Not Fighting Your Body

Living with All Forms of Adrenal Insufficiency

Not Fighting Your Body

Living With All Forms of Adrenal Insufficiency

© 2018 Lisa LaRue Baker

10 9 8 7 6 5 4 3 2 1

ISBN 978-1984911094

Third Childhood Publishing info@lisalaruemusic.com •
Topeka, Kansas, USA

Dedication

Dedicated with all of my love and sincere thanks to my husband, *John H. Baker*, whom has been by my side through every adrenal crisis, every doctor's appointment, every low cortisol episode resulting in the throwing of food he so kindly got me, and trying to explain my health and condition to nurses, doctors, friends, family and the public, since he's met me. A tireless advocate for not only me, but for those like me.

•

Also to *Dr. Jack Janway and Lynn Janway*; without their care I would likely not be alive, and without their mentoring, I likely would not have strived to learn about holistic and alternative medicine nor written this book.

•

And to my son, whom I love more than anything on this earth, and to whom I unfortunately passed on these terrible genes. *Spencer J. Snedden*, carry this book and my heart with you always. -Mom

Disclaimer

This book is not intended as a substitute for the medical advice of physicians. The reader should regularly consult a physician in matters relating to his/her health and particularly with respect to any symptoms that may require diagnosis or medical attention.

Table of Contents

Introduction

Adrenal Insufficiency is a nightmare. It is rare. It is a killer.

Adrenal Insufficiency is a 'real' disease – not a condition or syndrome, and has no cure. It is treatable, but even with treatment, emergencies will occur and they can be fatal without immediate intervention.

We hear a lot of buzz today about 'adrenal fatigue.' This book is not for you. If you believe you have a condition called 'adrenal fatigue' and try to treat yourself as if you had an actual Adrenal Insufficiency disease, you can make yourself incurably and fatally ill. If you believe you have 'adrenal fatigue' and think that people with Adrenal Insufficiency are the same as you, you could be risking their lives by not understanding the importance and immediacy of their illness. While many do not acknowledge the existence of 'adrenal fatigue' as there is no such 'disease,' to think that there is no such thing as Adrenal Insufficiency is a huge mistake. It would be analogous to thinking a person with diabetes is simply on a special diet because of weight.

John F. Kennedy is one famous person who had Addison's Disease, as is 1970's pop-singer Helen Reddy. But there are many people in our everyday world that are victims of Addison's, Congenital Adrenal Hyperplasia, and various forms of Adrenal Insufficiency. Many have died – some in their sleep – from an "Adrenal" or "Addisonian" Crisis.

This book is not meant in any way to replace medical treatment, but to help your body work with the medications and adapt the best it can to the new normal. Again, using diabetes as an analogy, if you were to be diagnosed with diabetes, you wouldn't think of taking your insulin but still eating candy, drinking pop and eating carbs, would you? You would make many changes to help the insulin work with your body, and to help your body be it's healthiest and best. *That* is what this book is all about.

Lisa LaRue Baker

Chapter One

Adrenal Insufficiency v Adrenal Deficiency
(AKA 'adrenal fatigue')

We hear about 'adrenal fatigue' on a daily basis. There are thousands of people in social media groups making appointments at various doctor's offices, and self-diagnosing with 'AF' because of being tired or showing 'symptoms' of Adrenal Insufficiency. This is dangerous for both the individual who feels something is wrong, as well as Adrenal Insufficiency patients.

If somebody treats themselves for Adrenal Insufficiency but doesn't have it, they can have fatal consequences if they discontinue the steroids they've been taking without proper weaning, since the adrenal glands quit making cortisol when you are artificially supplying the body with them. Suddenly stopping the medication will cause you to go into an Adrenal Crisis which can be fatal without immediate treatment. You cannot live without cortisol! That cannot be 'stressed' enough. Pun intended.

It is also dangerous to the Adrenal Insufficiency patient, because people start confusing their serious illness with a non-existent 'condition' and not take their treatment, care or emergencies seriously.

While a person may have numerous symptoms, it is important for an endocrinologist – a doctor who specializes in hormonal disorders – to assess your symptoms, history and order labs that they can interpret. Many illnesses have similar symptoms, and there is plenty of important information found by those trained in a physical exam and laboratory or even imaging analysis.

Adrenal Insufficiency is an endocrine disorder that occurs when the adrenal glands do not produce enough of certain hormones. These hormones are necessary for life. These hormones are typically cortisol and/or aldosterone. However, other hormones can be involved depending on if you have Addison's Disease, Secondary Adrenal Insufficiency or Congenital Adrenal Hyperplasia. There are forms of the illness that affect only cortisol, and there are also forms

1

of Adrenal Insufficiency that affect only aldosterone on a daily basis, but at a certain point in the crisis pathway, also involves cortisol. This is a very important thing to be aware of. A chart illustrating the latter is in Chapter 7.

What Are the Adrenal Glands?

An Italian anatomist called Bartolomeo Eustachi, is credited with the first description of the adrenal glands in 1563-4, but it was part of the papal library and did not receive public attention. The adrenal glands are named for their location – *ad*- is Latin for 'near,' and '*renes'* is Latin for 'kidney.' The term *Suprarenal*, a name given to the glands by Jean Riolan the Younger in 1629, means 'above' the kidney. This location, however, was not accepted until the 19th Century, as anatomists clarified the ductless nature of the glands and their secretory role. Prior to this, there was debate as to whether they were separate, or actually part of the kidney.

In 1855, English physician Thomas Addison published one of the most recognized works on the adrenals. In his *On the Constitutional and Local Effects of Disease of the Suprerenal Capsule*, Addison described what the French physician George Trousseau would later name Addison's disease... a condition of adrenal insufficiency and its related clinical manifestations. In 1894, English physiologists George Oliver and Edward Schafer studied the action of adrenal extracts, and observed their effects. In the following decades, several physicians experimented with extracts from the adrenal cortex to treat Addison's disease. Edward Calvin Kendall, Philip Hench and Tadeuz Reichstein were then awarded the 1950 *Nobel Prize* in physiology of medicine for their discoveries on the structure and effects of the adrenal hormones.

Scientists observed as early as the mid-nineteenth century that a lack of functional adrenal glands is incompatible with life. Further research categorized the effects of adrenal insufficiency into two distinct groups; those with electrolyte imbalance and those with altered carbohydrate metabolism. Progress was made in the 1930'a through the 1950's in understanding the hormones and how they were triggered, and isolated them from the adrenal cortex to characterize them for study. It was in 1949 when scientists discovered the efficacy of cortisol and ACTH in the treatment of

Rheumatoid Arthritis, and other anti-inflammatory illnesses and the medical world started using them in therapeutic applications.

Practical methods of plasma cortisol determination were then identified, and further research ensued. Ironically, the only treatments today for Adrenal Insufficiency are the same medications used at that time – simply replacements, but nothing to 'fix' the process of making these hormones.

Humans have two adrenal glands – one on top of each kidney, located in the back of the upper abdomen, or near the stomach. They are also known as the Suprarenal Glands, and consist of 2 parts. The inside layer is called the 'medulla,' and it produces the hormone epinephrine. People are familiar with epinephrine, as it is often referred to as the 'fight or flight' hormone, and is also a necessary injection for people who are allergic to bee stings or other allergies ('epi-pen' for example) or certain heart situations.

The outside layer of the adrenal is called the cortex, and makes important hormones that help the body to function normally. The main hormones are cortisol (a glucocorticoid) and aldosterone (a mineralocorticoid).

Cortisol

Cortisol affects almost every organ and tissue in the body, and scientists believe that it has possibly hundreds of effects in the body. This occurs because almost every cell has a cortisol receptor. Most importantly, it helps the body respond to stress – both physical and emotional. In this respect, it:

- maintains blood pressure and cardiovascular (heart and blood vessel) function
- mobilizes nutrients
- balances the effects of insulin in breaking down sugar for energy
- stimulates the liver to raise blood sugar
- regulates the metabolism of proteins, carbohydrates and fats
- assists with memory formulation
- supports a developing fetus during pregnancy
- slows the immune system's inflammatory response – this regulates how the body recognizes and defends itself against bacteria, viruses, and substances that appear foreign and harmful

The production of this hormone is precisely balanced, and is regulated by both the hypothalamus and the pituitary gland. The hypothalamus releases a hormone called Corticotropin-Releasing Hormone (CRH), which then signals the pituitary gland to send out another hormone called Adrenocorticotropic Hormone (ACTH) which then stimulates the adrenal to produce cortisol. Cortisol then signals back to both the pituitary gland and hypothalamus to decrease the trigger hormones. These actions have to happen within milliseconds, and you can easily understand how an imbalance can affect further production of cortisol, as well as many bodily functions necessary for life.

Aldosterone

Aldosterone helps maintain blood pressure and the balance of sodium and potassium in the blood and blood volume. People with Adrenal Insufficiency who do not produce enough aldosterone are known as 'salt wasting,' as when aldosterone production falls too low, the body loses too much sodium and retains too much potassium. The decrease of sodium in the blood leads to a drop in both blood volume (the amount of fluid in the blood) and blood pressure. This loss of fluid also leads to general dehydration. Third Spacing also occurs with low aldosterone, meaning dehydration while there is enough fluids to maintain hydration if they were 'moving.' Instead, they sit in interstitial areas of the body and don't move through cells. Too little sodium in the body can also cause a condition called hyponatremia, which includes feelings in incredible confusion, fatigue and causes muscle twitches and seizures. Too much potassium leads to a condition called hyperkalemia, which can cause irregular heartbeat, nausea, and a slow, weak and/or irregular pulse.

Due to the above, low aldosterone can cause dizziness, confusion, feeling faint, and as dehydration worsens the fluids drop more, blood pressure drops, and fainting can occur. At this point, cortisol starts being expended, as well, to try and keep the body from shutting down fully - which leads to coma. If no intervention is made, the patient can potentially die, or revive with severe brain or organ failure and/or damage. The Pathways to Adrenal Crisis chart in chapter 7 illustrates this action.

More about Adrenal Crisis in chapter 7, perhaps the most important chapter in this book.

Dehydroepiandrosterone (DHEA)

DHEA is another hormone produced by the adrenal glands. This hormone is used by the body to manufacture sex hormones including androgens and estrogen. Those who suffer Adrenal Insufficiency may also suffer in inadequate DHEA production. Although healthy men derive most androgens from the testes and healthy women derive most of their estrogen from the ovaries, women and adolescent girls may experience various symptoms from DHEA insufficiency which includes loss of pubic hair, dry skin, a reduced interest in sex, and depression. NIH cites DHEA deficiency as a form of Adrenal Insufficiency, as well.

Addison's Disease

Addison's Disease is rare – only one in 100,000 people are believed to have it. Addison's is considered "Primary Adrenal Insufficiency," which occurs when the adrenal cortex is damaged and doesn't produce its hormones in adequate quantities. The failure of adrenal glands to produce adrenocortical hormones is most commonly the result of the body attacking itself, or 'autoimmune disease.' Other damage which can cause adrenal gland failure may include:

- infections of the adrenal glands
- cancer of the adrenal glands
- tuberculosis
- bleeding of the adrenal glands – which can present as an Adrenal Crisis without any preceding symptoms

Addison's, or Primary Adrenal Insufficiency, is basically caused by the total or near total destruction of the adrenal glands and usually results in severe deficiency of both cortisol and aldosterone.

Secondary Adrenal Insufficiency

Adrenal Insufficiency can also occur if the pituitary gland is diseased. As stated above, the pituitary gland makes a hormone called Adrenocorticotropic Hormone (ACTH), which stimulates the adrenal cortex to produce its hormones. Inadequate production of ACTH can lead to insufficient production of hormones normally produced by the adrenal glands, even though the adrenals aren't damaged. This is termed "Secondary Adrenal Insufficiency." Secondary Adrenal Insufficiency can be caused by diseases of the hypothalamus and/or pituitary, such as pituitary tumors, craniopharyngiomas, surgery to remove a tumor, radiation therapy to the pituitary, cysts in the pituitary, and some inflammatory diseases.

Secondary Adrenal Insufficiency can also occur when people who take corticosteroids for treatment of chronic conditions, such as asthma or arthritis, abruptly stop taking the corticosteroids. This can also happen to people who self-diagnose themselves with 'adrenal fatigue' and try to treat themselves as if they had Adrenal Insufficiency. These medications include cortisone, hydrocortisone, prednisone, prednisolone, dexamethasone, as well as intravenous, intramuscular, inhaled and topical steroids. They all have an effect on ACTH because the pituitary is producing this hormone in response to the body's need for cortisol – when the cells in the pituitary recognize any of these drugs, they pick up the signal that cortisol is present and therefore produce less ACTH. This can be temporary, prolonged, or permanent depending on the strength of the medication, and the length of time they were taken.

If the Secondary Adrenal Insufficiency is due to these reasons, there is normally the absence of normal stimulation of cortisol production from a lack of ACTH. While this results in a partial or total deficiency of cortisol, there is often a normal, or near normal, production of aldosterone. As always, there are exceptions.

Adrenalectomy

A cause of total lack of adrenal hormones is due to an adrenalectomy – the removal of one or both glands. Obviously, if both glands are removed, no adrenal hormones are produced. Adrenal glands can be removed due to tumors, which are usually found during medical imaging, and often when causes for Cushing's Syndrome or Disease are being explored. (Cushing's is the illness that results due to an *overproduction* of cortisol.) Most often, adrenal tumors are benign adenomas, and carcinomas are very rare. Another type of adrenal tumor is a Pheochromocytoma, tumors of the medulla that arise from chromaffin cells. These tumors can produce a variety of nonspecific symptoms including sweating, anxiety, headache, and heart palpitations. Signs can include hypertension and tachycardia.

Congenital Adrenal Hyperplasia

Congenital Adrenal Hyperplasia, or CAH, is a disease present at birth (congenital) in which mutations of enzymes that produce steroid hormones result in a glucocorticoid deficiency and malfunction of the negative feedback loop of the HPA Axis (Hypothalmic-Pituitary-Adrenal). In this axis, cortisol inhibits the release of CRH and ACTH, hormones that in-turn stimulate the production of cortisol. Since cortisol can't be made, the hormones are released in high quantities and stimulate production of other hormones, instead. Although an extremely rare disease, the most common form of CAH is due to 21-hydroxylase deficiency. This enzyme is necessary for production of both aldosterone and cortisol, but not androgens. Because of this, ACTH stimulation of the adrenal cortex induces the release of excessive amounts of adrenal androgens (sex hormones, such as testosterone), which can lead to the development of ambiguous genitalia present at birth and secondary sex characteristics. The mutation is found on 6p21.3 as part of the HLA complex, and results from a unique mutation with two highly homologous near-copies in series consisting of an active gene (CYP21A) and an inactive pseudogene (CYP21P). Mutant alleles result from recombination between the active and pseudo genes. An even further variability depends on the degree of enzyme inefficiency produced by the specific alleles each patient has. Some alleles result in more severe degrees of enzyme efficiency. Severe degrees of inefficiency produce changes in the fetus, and problems in prenatal or perinatal life. However, milder degrees are usually associated with excessive –or deficient- sex hormone effects in childhood or adolescence, and the mildest form can sometimes only interfere with ovulation and fertility in adults. Synthesis of cortisol shares steps with synthesis of aldosterone, so people with CAH have varying degrees of salt-wasting, as well. Female infants with classic CAH are born with ambiguous genitalia due to high concentrations of androgens *in utero*. Less severely affected females may present with early puberty, and young women may present with polycystic ovarian syndrome, absent periods and hirsutism. Males with classic CAH generally have no signs of CAH at birth, but some may present with dark pigmentation of the genitals and possible penile enlargement. The age of diagnosis for males depends on the severity of aldosterone deficiency. In rarer forms of CAH, males are under-masculinized, and females generally have no signs or symptoms at birth.

Classic 21-hydroxylase deficiency typically causes 17α-hydroxyprogesterone blood levels >242 nmol/L. Salt-wasting patients tend to have higher 17α-hydroxyprogesterone levels than non-salt-wasting patients. In mild cases, 17α-hydroxyprogesterone may not be elevated in a particular random blood sample, but it will rise during a corticotropin stimulation test.

There are several other autosomal recessive forms of CAH, including 11β-hydroxylase, 3β –HSD, 17α-hydroxylase, and lipoid. These forms are very different from each other, and some involve aldosterone excess and sex hormone deficiency.

Currently in the United States and over 40 other countries, every child born is screened for 21-hydroxylase CAH at birth. This test will detect elevated levels of 17-hydroxy-progesterone (17-OHP). This enables early detection of CAH, and newborns can avoid an adrenal crisis during the first week or two of life, and be put on medication at the earliest date.

Since CAH is a recessive gene, both the mother and father must be recessive carriers of CAH for a child to have CAH. Due to advances in modern medicine, couples with the genes have an option to prevent CAH in their offspring through preimplantation genetic diagnosis. In this process, the egg is fertilized outside of the woman's body and on the 3rd day, when the embryo has developed from one cell to about 4 to 6 cells, one of those cells is removed from the embryo without harming the embryo. The embryo continues to grow until day 5 when it is either frozen or implanted into the mother.

Hypoaldosteronism

A form of adrenal hyperplasia that primarily affects aldosterone is called Hypoaldosteronism, and there are several forms of this illness, as well. Causes of hypoaldsteronism can be both acquired and inherited (less common). *Isolated Hypoaldosteronism* is the condition of having lowered aldosterone without corresponding changes in cortisol.

Primary Aldosterone deficiency can be caused by
•CAH 21 and 11β but not 17)
•Aldosterone synthase deficiency

Secondary Aldosterone Deficiency can be caused by diseases of the pituitary of hypothalamus, and Hyporeninemic Hypo-aldosteronism, due to decreased angiotensin 2 production as well as intra-adrenal dysfunction, can be caused by
•Renal dysfunction – most commonly diabetic neuropathy
•NSAIDs
•angiotensin inhibitors
•heparin therapy
•critical illness
•Ciclosporin

Aldosterone Resistance can be caused by inhibitors of the epithelial sodium channel (potassium-sparing diuretics, trimethoprim, pentamidine).

Congenital Hypoaldosteronism/Visser-Cost Syndrome

Congenital hypoaldosteronism due to an isolated aldosterone biosynthesis defect is rare, and is a defect of the terminal aldosterone biosynthesis. Aldosterone biosynthesis requires 11 beta-hydroxylation of 11-deoxycorticosterone to form corticosterone, hydroxylation at potision C-18 to form 18-hydroxycorticosterone (18-OHB), and finally oxidation at position C-18. One single cytochrome P450 enzyme (P450 aldo) catalyzes all three reactions and the coding gene is termed CYP11B2. Two inborn errors of terminal aldosterone biosynthesis characterized by overproduction of corticosterone and deficient synthesis of aldosterone have been described. Corticosterone methyl oxidase deficiency type I (CMO I) is distinguished by decreased production of 18-OHB while CMO II is characterized by overproduction of 18-OHB and an elevated ratio of 18-OHB to aldosterone. Both disorders are inherited by an autosomal recessive trait and cause salt wasting and failure to thrive in early infancy. So far, scientists and researchers have discovered three different mutations within the CYPIIB2 gene in patients with P450 aldosterone deficiency.

This disorder is characterized by excessive amounts of sodium released in the urine, or salt-wasting, along with insufficient release of potassium in the urine, usually beginning in the first few weeks of life. This imbalance leads to low levels of sodium and high levels of potassium in the blood. Individuals with corticosterone methyloxidase deficiency can also have high levels of acid in the blood (metabolic acidosis). The hyponatremia, hyperkalemia, and metabolic acidosis associated with corticosterone methyloxidase deficiency can cause nausea, vomiting, dehydration, low blood pressure, extreme fatigue, and muscle weakness. Infants often experience failure to thrive. Severe cases of corticosterone methyloxidase deficiency can result in seizures and coma and can be life-threatening. In some cases, the disorder can become milder or disappear by adulthood, although this is not always the case.

Adrenal Fatigue

Adrenal fatigue is not a recognized illness, nor syndrome. It is a 'theory' and 'concept' that has no diagnostic testing to verify its existence. All the labs for adrenal illness can be run, but there will be no differentials to show the adrenals are 'fatigued.' I can't deny, however, that there is no such thing as 'adrenal *deficiency*,' especially in the case of Secondary Adrenal Insufficiency, where they are damaged. You can't just be well one day, and the next have full-blown Adrenal Insufficiency, but you will –hopefully- notice changes that allow your doctor to diagnose Adrenal Insufficiency in it's early stages so you can begin treatment and hopefully prevent an Adrenal Crisis as much as possible.

Adrenal fatigue is a term that has been given to a collection of symptoms that are non-specific. Everything from insomnia, digestive problems, and fatigue itself has been attributed to it. It is an unproven theory that the adrenal glands become unstable and unable to 'keep up' with chronic stress. While it is quite possible you have an illness, or you need medical attention, 'adrenal fatigue' self-diagnosis and various theories of curing it, are dangerous. As stated above, you can actually *cause* yourself to develop incurable and lifethreatening Adrenal Insufficiency, and you can also cause others to not take actual Adrenal Insufficiency seriously, thinking the person is just referring to 'adrenal fatigue.' Lastly, you could be ignoring another actual illness that may need attention and treatment.

Adrenal fatigue was first described by James Wilson in 1998. Wilson is an alternative medicine doctor, and many people have used this to ignore *any* alternative medicine doctor, whether a naturopath, a homeopath, an herbalist or other. This is NOT true. There are many reputable alternative medicine doctors throughout the world who recognize that actual medical conditions can be incurable, but will work with allopathic doctors (MD's, etc.) to give the patient a full range of care – oftentimes resulting in less medication needed, better quality of life, and less medical emergencies. Under no circumstance would a reputable alternative doctor or practitioner recommend that a person quit taking necessary-for-life medication! If you encounter such a practitioner, run! Most reputable practitioners will, however, recognize adrenal distress and recommend you see an endocrinologist for proper testing, diagnosis, and treatment.

Sources used in this chapter:
Hormones of the Adrenal Cortex, Lorraine I. McKay and John A. Cidlowski, PhD
Holland-Frei Cancer Medicine, 6th Edition
MayoClinic.org
Wikipedia
Pediatr Res. 1996 Mar; 39(3):554-60
Congenital Hypoaldosteronism: The Visser-Cost Syndrome Revisited, Peter M. Sippell, as published by NOH
US National Library of Medicine, NIH
Niddk.nih.com
Medicalnewstoday.com

Chapter Two

Diagnosis

One of the most important, and most frustrating, things to pay attention to is getting a proper diagnosis. Lack of education and knowledge of the illness itself makes it hard to get proper attention from doctors and practitioners. The suggested steps to diagnosis are:

•recognizing symptoms
•discussing the symptoms with your primary care physician or regular practitioner
•depending on how your insurance works, get a referral to an endocrinologist (a physician who specializes in hormonal diseases)
•familiarize yourself with the tests that may occur to investigate the diagnosis you are seeking
•understanding the instructions for testing and following the prep requirements
•following up with obtaining copies of your test results, and ask for interpretation from the endocrinologist, your primary care physician, and another physician should be you choose to, or be able to, have a second opinion

Depending on your situation, there may be other options available to you. There are companies online such as WalkInLabs, who allow you to order lab tests and they then provide you with a doctor-signed order to take to their designated laboratory facility. You can then get your labs completed and the results without a doctor's order (other than the one the company provides). The prices are relatively inexpensive. If you do not have the ability to interpret these results, you can also look into telemedicine. Provide these results to the telemedicine physician, and get an opinion from them. You can then take the notes from the telemed physician and the lab results to your primary care physician, or to an endocrinologist and ask them to explore further. Some people choose to do this, because it gives their suspicions validation where oftentimes GP's will not consider the patient's opinions or ideas. Validation from labs and other physicians gives them reason to explore, and also shows them your knowledge and seriousness.

Below is the list of symptoms you should document if you begin to notice them and are concerned about Adrenal Insufficiency. When documenting them, be sure to make notes of time of day, what you had eaten, what activities you were doing, etc. At the end of each section is a list of tests you can expect your doctor to recommend, or that you can ask about if they do not.

Primary Adrenal Insufficiency
- Extreme chronic fatigue
- Decreased appetite
- Weight loss
- Hyperpigmentation (darkening of skin)
- Low blood pressure – frequently, or upon standing (orthostatic)
- Near fainting or fainting
- Salt craving
- Hypoglycemia (low blood sugar)
- Nausea, vomiting, diarrhea
- Abdominal and/or flank pain
- Joint and muscle pain; muscle weakness
- Irritability, anxiety, depression
- Body hair loss
- Frequent headaches
- Irregular or absent menstrual periods
- Low Sodium levels in blood
- High potassium levels in blood
- Loss of sexual desire in women

Acute Adrenal Insufficiency is also suspected in the presence of unexplained catecholamine-resistant hypotention.

Diagnosis: Your doctor will do a physical exam and take a complete history, and will ask if you have a family history of Addison's Disease. The physical exam will give her a chance to look for changes in skin color, signs of dehydration, and check your blood pressure and heart.

14

Blood tests will be taken to check your cortisol, ACTH, aldosterone and electrolytes (such as potassium and sodium). Your doctor should also order an ACTH Stimulation Test to see how your hormone levels react to stress. Imaging may be ordered as well, such as a CT Scan or MRI to look for damage to the adrenal glands.

Other tests can include 11-Deoxycortisol, Dexamethasone Suppression, Adrenal Antibody, and 21-Hydroxylase Antibody.

Secondary Adrenal Insufficiency
    Same as above, EXCEPT
    •Hyperpigmentation (darkening of skin)
    •Low sodium levels in blood
    •High potassium levels in blood

Profound weight loss and loss of appetite are major symptoms.

If you have had any of the procedures or injuries listed in chapter 1 that can cause Secondary Adrenal Insufficiency and experience any of these symptoms, you should contact your physician immediately.

Diagnosis: A physical exam along with a medical history will begin the investigation; be sure you take all records of injuries and procedures. If your doctor agrees to test for Adrenal Insufficiency, they will check your blood cortisol and ACTH levels. They 'may' check aldosterone and electrolyte levels, and they may also do imaging of the adrenals, pituitary and/or hypothalamus such as a CT scan or MRI. This is to see if there are signs of damage or trauma in the brain, such as a tumor. In secondary adrenal insufficiency, aldosterone and electrolytes 'should' be normal, while cortisol and ACTH will be low. Your doctor may give you infusions of ACTH for 2 days in a row. It is likely that your adrenal glands will make cortisol by the end of the second treatment, even if you have problems with the hypothalamus or pituitary. If it is found you are not making cortisol due to deficient ACTH production, your doctor will begin treatment.

Other tests can include 11-Deoxycortisol, Dexamethasone Suppression,

Congenital Adrenal Hyperplasia

While Congenital Adrenal Hyperplasia is often diagnosed at birth due to screening, there are some states and countries that do not mandate these tests. In addition, there are people who may have late-onset CAH who do not present until early adulthood, who were not tested at birth. Therefore, watching for symptoms is still important as a young adult, and should be reported to a physician for further investigation.

- Frequent vomiting (due to salt wasting)
- Dehydration (due to salt wasting)
- Low Blood Pressure (due to salt wasting)
- Syncope (near fainting or fainting) (due to salt wasting)
- In males, extreme virilization, but no sperm
- Ambiguous genitalia in some females (due to high androgens)
- Early pubic hair and rapid growth in childhood (due to high androgens)
- Excessive facial hair (due to high androgens)
- Failure or delayed puberty
- Menstrual irregularity or absence of menses (due to high androgens)
- Infertility due to anovulation (due to high androgens)
- Enlarged clitoris and shallow vagina (due to high androgens)
- Undervirilization in XY males resulting in apparently female external genitalia
- Premature phallic enlargement in the absence of testicular enlargement
- Hypogonadism in females

Diagnosis: While screening-at-birth is mandatory in most states and numerous countries, it is not everywhere. An older person with late-onset may have missed the window of screening/testing, as well. Pre-natal screening in pregnancies where parents are known carriers of CAH mutations can also be accomplished. Newborn screening programs for 21-hydroxylase deficiency should be encouraged as they may be lifesaving in an affected male infant who would otherwise be undetected due to no physical characteristics such as ambiguous genitalia, until presentation with a salt-wasting crisis.

If a doctor suspects 21-hydroxylase Congenital Adrenal Hyperplasia due to inadequate production of cortisol, aldosterone, or both in the presence of accumulation of excess concentrations of precursor hormones, typical diagnosis can consist of:

Testing of 17-hydroxy-progesterone (17-OHP), which may be run several times due to a high false positive rate. The doctor will also test urinary prenanetriol. 24-hour urinary testing for elevated 17-ketosteroids will also be checked.

11-beta-hydroxylase deficiency CAH will be confirmed by testing for excess concentrations of 11-deoxycortisol and deoxycorticosterone, or by an elevation in the ratio of 24-hour urinary tetrahydrocompound S to tetrahydrocompound F, in addition to 24-hour urinary 17-ketosteroids.

Salt wasting forms of CAH are confirmed by low aldosterone concentrations, low sodium, high potassium, and elevated plasma renin activity. However, hypertensive forms of adrenal hyperplasia such as 11-beta-hydroxylase deficiency and 17-alpha-hydroxylase deficiency are associated with suppressed plasma renin activity, and often low potassium.

Mild forms of adrenal hyperplasia, such as non-classic forms of 21-hydroxylase deficiency and nonclassic 3-beta-hydroxysteroid dehydrogenase deficiency often require a Cortrosyn (synthetic corticotropin) stimulation test to demonstrate the abnormal accumulation of precursor steroids.

While imaging of the adrenal glands are usually not useful in evaluating patients with suspected adrenal hyperplasia, CT scans *can* be useful in excluding bilateral adrenal hemorrhage in patients who are showing signs of Adrenal Crisis without other outward symptoms.

Pelvic ultrasound may be performed on infants with ambiguous genitalia to demonstrate a uterus or renal anomalies, and urogenitography is often helpful in defining the anatomy of the internal genitalia. A karyotype is essential in the evaluation of an infant with ambiguous genitalia to establish the patient's chromosomal sex. Genetic testing is rarely necessary to diagnose classic forms of adrenal hyperplasia, but is essential for genetic counseling and prenatal diagnosis of adrenal hyperplasia. Lastly, a bone-age study is useful in evaluating a child who develops precocious pubic hair, clitoromegaly, or accelerated linear growth.

Patients who have these symptoms because of adrenal hyperplasia have advanced skeletal maturation.

Lipoid adrenal hyperplasia will show lipoid deposits in the adrenal cortical cells due to a deficiency of StAR. Lipoid deposits are thought to represent cholesterol esters that have accumulated from the inability of the cell to transport cholesterol into the mitochondria.

Other tests may include Androstenedione, DHEA, 17-Hydroxypregnenolone, Progesterone, 17-Hydroxyprogesterone, and Testosterone.

Hypoaldosteronism
- Hyperkalemia (high potassium)
- Mild anion-gap metabolic acidosis
- Low sodium
- High potassium
- Aldosterone – Renin ratio
- Plasma renin activity

Hyporeninemic hypoaldosteronism is commonly seen in patients with renal insufficiency, such as diabetic kidney disease, chronic tubulointerstitial disease, or glomerulonephritis, and those that take certain medications such as non-steroidal anti-inflammatory drugs and calcineurin inhibitors.

Doctors will look for the use of angiotensin inhibitors, ACE inhibitors, ARBs and direct renin inhibitors as well as heparin therapy. Heparin has a direct toxic effect on the adrenal zona glomerulosa cells which leads to a reduction in plasma aldosterone concentration.

If the patient has had a critical illness resulting in a decreased adrenal production of aldosterone and stress-induced hypersecretion of ACTH, this can diminish aldosterone synthesis by diverting substrate to the production of cortisol.

If the patient does not have Primary or Secondary Adrenal Insufficiency or CAH, CYPIIB2 will be genetically checked to see if there is a deficiency in the enzyme required for aldosterone synthesis. There have been cases of patients who have non-salt wasting Adrenal Insufficiency, who *are* salt wasting due to a deficiency of this enzyme.

Patients who use potassium-sparing diuretics such as spironolactone, eplerenone, or amiloride, and certain antibiotics such as trimethoprim or pentamidine, will be evaluated to see if this is the cause for low aldosterone.

If the patient has signs and symptoms of low aldosterone by has marked elevations of plasma aldosterone, they will be investigated for Pseudohypoaldosteronism Type 1. There is an autosomal recessive form, and an autosomal dominant or sporadic form.

Presenting with an Adrenal Crisis
ADRENAL CRISIS IS AN IMMEDIATE MEDICAL EMERGENCY.

Some patients are not diagnosed until they present with a life-threatening Adrenal Crisis. If any of the Adrenal Insufficiency diseases have not been suspected, it can be quite mysterious to medical personnel what is wrong. If the patient is a child that has not been screened for Congenital Adrenal Hyperplasia, they should be treated for adrenal crisis if showing symptoms before labs are drawn to seek diagnosis. There is no time to spare!

Adrenal Crisis is a life-threatening condition that occurs when there is not enough cortisol – or when there is a salt-wasting crisis which crosses over in the pathway of events to use up cortisol.

Symptoms after Diagnosis

If the patient has already been diagnosed with an Adrenal Insufficiency disease, and they are
- ill
- injured
- fever
- vomiting
- diarrhea
- traumatic event
- extraordinary activity
- faint

they should take extra 'stress doses' of their steroids, and extra salt or electrolytes if salt wasting. Adrenal crisis can occur from the following:

- Addison's Disease, other Adrenal Insufficiency diseases
- You've been dehydrated
- Infection or other stress

Symptoms of Adrenal Crisis include but are not limited to:
- Abdominal or flank pain
- Confusion
- Loss of consciousness or coma
- Dehydration
- Dizziness, lightheadedness or feeling faint
- Severe weakness
- Headache
- High fever
- Low blood pressure
- High blood pressure that drops upon standing
- Nausea and vomiting
- Rapid heart rate
- Rapid respiratory rate
- Slow, sluggish movement and speaking
- Unusual and excessive sweating on face or palms

REMEMBER! In adrenal crisis, you will need intravenous or intramuscular hydrocortisone immediately, even before seeking medical care. It is important to carry your emergency injection at all times, and those that are around you often know where it is and how to use it. Once you have begun receiving medical care, you may also receive intravenous fluids if you have low blood pressure. After getting your emergency injection, you will need further treatment and monitoring. If infection of another medical problem caused your crisis, you will need treatment for that, as well.

SHOCK may occur if treatment is not provided early, and it can be lifethreatening.

You will also need to increase your steroid dosage and have a high-dose injection if you are very ill, or prior to any surgery or certain procedures. If you are having surgery talk to the surgeon as well as the anesthesiologist, and have orders from your endocrinologist.

Resources for this chapter:

Web MD
John Hopkins POC-It Guides
National Institute of Diabetes and Digestive and Kidney Diseases, US Department of Health and Human Services
Medscape
Medlineplus.gov
Quest Diagnostics
Pocket Reference for ICU Staff, Critical Care Medicine Services, Tripler Army Medical Center, Honolulu, HI

Chapter Three

What to Expect From Your Doctor

So you've been diagnosed. Now what? There are several things to expect from your doctor; first, the standard patient's rights, and second, what he or she would do for you specifically, as an adrenal insufficiency patient.

Both are equally important.

As far as patient's rights, some are guaranteed to you by federal law, and some of them are protected by state laws. Many health care facilities often have a patient's bill of rights. Check with the Office Manager at your provider's office to get copies of the laws and bill of rights that apply. Some larger facilities have a patient advocate that can address these questions, or your state's Health Department can also provide information.

Once you are diagnosed with Adrenal Insufficiency, you should expect your doctor to explain to you the lab results, and his or her interpretation of them – the diagnosis. This is why it was important to be familiar with the tests that should be ordered when you first present for diagnosis, so you can ask pertinent questions. Especially if you feel the doctor is not explaining well, or giving you complete information. Ask every question you can, and expect an answer. If there are any questions your doctor cannot answer, ask if there is another provider in the practice that can answer these questions for you.

If the diagnosis was given by your Primary Care Provider, you should expect the doctor to refer you to an Endocrinologist. An endocrinologist is a doctor who specializes in the endocrine – or hormonal – system. Some insurance companies, or even regions, have limitations. Try to ensure that the endocrinologist you are being referred to does not specialize in Diabetes, or Reproductive Endocrinology, but rather in Adrenal Diseases, which can be very important in your treatment and care. If your doctor is hesitant about putting you on steroids (hydrocortisone, for example) for low cortisol or a mineralocorticoid (fludrocortisone) for low aldosterone before seeing your endocrinologist, ask them to reconsider *and* make sure that whomever is making your referral marks it as urgent – it *is* urgent that you get on your treatment as soon as possible to avoid having a lifethreatening Adrenal Crisis!

When you arrive at the endocrinologist's office, make sure you take your notes with you regarding your diagnosis, an extra copy of your lab reports in case they have gotten lost in transport from the other office, and a list of any questions you may have – it's easy to forget important questions when you get in the exam room! Ask the same questions you asked the Primary Care Physician, even if you felt you got a good answer before.

Ask the endocrinologist what medications he or she is prescribing, and ask about dosing – it is important that your doctor explain to you the best dosing for your situation, and ask them if 'circadian' dosing is appropriate for you. Circadian dosing follows the natural rhythm of the human body's production and release of cortisol, and can be very effective. Also ask the doctor if a cortisol pump may be appropriate for you. It is similar to an insulin pump that are prescribed for Diabetics. Some of these questions may be inappropriate at the time, or even for your case, but it will let your endocrinologist know that you are very aware of adrenal illnesses and treatment.

If you are salt-wasting and require fludrocortisone, make sure that you speak to the doctor about salt intake, as well. Salt is extremely important to the human body, and some physicians highly recommend additional sodium (salt) even though you are taking fludrocortisone. Ask them for recommendations for those times your blood pressure starts getting low, you feel faint, or it's especially hot and humid outside.

You should also expect your doctor to prescribe an emergency injection for you to carry at all times. This is extremely important!! It may be Solu-Cortef, Dexamethasone, or even Betamethasone, but be sure the doctor or their assistant explains to you when to use it, and how to use it. Make sure you have a family member or friend with you who is normally close at hand in your life, so they know how to use it when you are unable to. This injection can save your life. Lastly, make sure there are enough refills on your prescription that you won't run out. If you happen to have insurance that will not cover these injections, do *not* choose to go without! This injection can save your life, and at the time of this writing, the average injection cost is $16.00. A very low cost to save your life, so don't be bothered if it is not covered by insurance.

You should expect your doctor to answer any of your questions, and to provide a phone number for their assistant should you have further questions, and instructions for how to contact the office in case of emergency. The latter is very important, in case you are in an accident, or need to go to the emergency room – the attending providers may need to speak to your endocrinologist for orders as soon as possible.

There is one other thing you should expect from your doctor, but it may not be automatically provided. This is an emergency instructions/orders letter. There is a copy in the "In Case of Emergency" chapter of this book; your doctor may wish to modify it, or simply sign the copy in this book, so that you can keep this book with you at all times so all information is handy in case of an accident, or you are unconscious.

Many, many emergency services and even emergency rooms do not have protocols for Adrenal Crisis. The staff are not even trained to recognize one. It is even increasingly difficult to get an anesthesiologist to recognize the need for a 100 mg Solu-Cortef shot when you are going to have a procedure or surgery. One has to wonder what kind of training the practitioner and support staff receives, when most veterinarians even give a dexamethasone shot automatically when doing surgery or major procedures. With that being said, you should always ask your provider to give specific orders when surgery or a major procedure is being done, *and* to provide you with an emergency letter that you can show or give in any situation.

You should expect your provider's office to always respond to your calls and emails. Adrenal Insufficiency patients often have emergency situations – whether it is an accident, or a viral infection, or news of death of a loved one, and you need answers immediately if you feel you might go into crisis.

Most experienced Adrenal Insufficiency patients say, "shoot first, ask questions later." In other words, when in doubt – inject.

You should also expect your primary care provider to work with your endocrinologist! If you can't get ahold of the endocrinologist, the primary should be familiar enough with your case and have adequate notes to call in emergency prescriptions, advise emergency personnel, or to see you to check your vitals and prescribe in-office fluids, if needed.

You should expect your physician to be familiar with not only diagnostic testing, but labs to check as maintenance. The previous chapter lists the tests which should be conducted to investigate each variation of Adrenal Insufficiency.

Lastly and most importantly, you should expect your doctor to be a part of your team. You depend on them.

Chapter Four

More to Taking Care of Yourself Than That!

When a person who was not born with a form of Adrenal Insufficiency receives a diagnosis, oftentimes today, they will search the internet for more information, and oftentimes, the new AI patient will find information that states "once medication is started, life continues normally." Unfortunately, this is rarely true.

Your body requires a certain amount of cortisol each day, on a circadian rhythm, to function. Just to function. The body normally creates a surge of cortisol in milliseconds when needed – injury, accident, etc. This is in addition to the amount needed just for the body to function. So even though you are taking oral amounts to 'function,' we have to worry about the 'extra' in the case of injury, illness, and all of the other things. This is called 'stress dosing.'

Make sure your physician prescribes enough 'extra' steroid that you can stress dose! Your provider will be able to give you directions and guidelines for stress dosing, but every person and every situation is different. One word of caution with steroids! DO NOT quit taking them 'cold turkey,' and don't stress dose for more than 2 or 3 days without 'weaning down' back to your regular dosage. This can be deadly, and cause an Adrenal Crisis, due to the body becoming quickly dependent on and used to a different amount of cortisol. Repeat, DO NOT do this!

If you use steroids on a regular basis, the HPA (hypothalamic-pituitary-adrenal) axis may be suppressed, and the adrenal glands not respond appropriately. The adrenals will react the same way during times of stress such as surgery. Regular use of extra steroids can also cause impaired wound healing, increased friability of skin, superficial blood vessels, and other tissues. Simple, everyday things like removing medical tape, can damage and tear your skin. You also have an increased risk of fractures, infections, gastrointestinal hemorrhage, or ulcer. This is with extremely high, more-than-needed doses, however. Taking replacements doses to cover what you *should* be producing, should not affect you this way.

It is imperative that you take extra steroids when having surgery. Surgery is one of the most potent activators of the HPA axis. Plasma ACTH concentrations should raise, in the healthy person, at the moment of incision, and during surgery., with the greatest secretion of both ACTH and cortisol occurs during the reversal of anesthesia, when your breathing tube is removed, and in the immediate postoperative recovery period. It is also important to note that plasma ACTH and cortisol responses to surgery can also be reduced by opiate drugs. In general, the adrenal gland in a healthy person produces about 50 mg/day during a minor procedure (the normal base rate is 8 to 10 mg per day), while 75 to 100 mg a day are produced with major surgery. Amazingly, natural cortisol secretion rate can reach 200 to 500 mg per day with severe stress, but secretion rates greater than 200 mg per day are rare.

Always keep a stash available for weaning down in case you can't get a refill, due to availability or natural disaster. Speaking of natural disaster, always keep a supply of steroids, mineralocorticoids and emergency injections in your earthquake kit, basement, or wherever you seek shelter in case of an emergency. Even your purse, in case you get stalled away from home or there is a fire.

When you are salt wasting (low aldosterone), fludrocortisone is necessary to balance water, salt and potassium, as is extra salt. But there are lots of factors that can change your dosage of this medication, as well. Humidity levels, high temperature, or even drops in humidity or temperature can change the fluid levels in your body. Often, if fluids and electrolytes quit moving, a person will experience 'third spacing' where the fluids just 'sit' in the interstitial spaces between the cells, and not move 'through' cells or to the parts of the body, including making blood volume, like it should. In these cases, you have enough fluid, but you become dehydrated due to third spacing! It is important to not only have your fludrocortisone, but sodium, magnesium, and other electrolytes to try and keep fluids moving. More about this in other chapters.

This means you have to watch for times you need extra steroids, or stress dosing, every single day. As you get more experience with your new normal, you will learn to predict when you will need to stress dose, thus making it possible to do so *before* your body takes a beating from low cortisol, starts going into crisis, or maybe goes *into* crisis. Sometimes these are 'good' stresses. A birthday party for your 5 year old which requires you to make a cake, decorate the house, entertain 14 other 5 year olds, etc. Or perhaps it's your wedding day.

The recommended times for stress dosing are:

- Fever of 101 F or more (or equivalent, based on your normal body temperature)
- Diarrhea
- Vomiting
- Ear infection
- Strep Throat
- Pneumonia
- Bronchitis
- Broken Bone
- Sprain or strain
- Serious injury/accident
- Surgical procedure
- Immunizations
- Other times based on your history and experience.

Some doctors recommend doubling your normal dose for 3 days. However, if you take the oral stress dose and vomit within 20-30 minutes, take another stress dose. If you vomit again, you will need to take an emergency injection. (*Once you take your injection, it is very important to go to the emergency room WITHIN 4 HOURS for medical treatment. Tell the emergency doctors you have Adrenal Insufficiency, and give them a copy of your Emergency Orders from your doctor. Tell them what medicines you take for AI regularly, when your last dose was, and that you have injected with your emergency injection.*)

If you are stress dosing *without* having to take an emergency injection, and are ill for more than 3 days, you should contact or visit your provider.

You also need to be aware of weather, and amount of activity, how much salt you intake, and the dosage of fludrocortisone on a daily basis, and compare it with your blood pressure. For example, if it gets exceptionally hot outside, and very humid, and you are outside a lot or don't have air conditioning, you should pay particular attention to your blood pressure. If it is dropping low, or it drops when you stand up, you need to take a larger dose of fludrocortisone, or you need to take some salt – either through a salt tablet, eating an apple with salt on it, eating a pickle, or some other way. Try to avoid generally unhealthy salty snacks, such as potato chips, and don't fall for 'pickle-flavored' snacks. Just because they 'taste' like pickles, doesn't mean they have the sodium content or other nutrients of pickles. There are other suggestions for this elsewhere in this book, but be aware that you need to be aware of climate, environment, and electrolyte intake on a daily basis.

Low Cortisol

After diagnosis and starting treatment, you may notice times where you seem to be reverting to your condition previous to diagnosis. Perhaps these are not 'stress dose' times, but maybe you are needing a stronger dose of steroids, or perhaps the same amount but taken in smaller increments at different times, or more on a circadian rhythm. Signs of low cortisol should be reported to your endocrinologist as soon as possible to avoid crisis point. Refer to the list of low cortisol symptoms at the beginning of this book, or the list of symptoms you reported when you were first diagnosed.

Too Much Cortisol?

If you stress dose 'too often,' or are on too high of a replacement dose of steroids, you may start to notice signs and symptoms of Cushing's Syndrome.

Cushing's Syndrome is different than Cushing's Disease, as the disease is normally caused by tumors or other maladies, while the syndrome is usually caused by reversible behavior, such as too much steroid dosing. Stress dosing one or two times too many during an illness, or several times a year, should not cause this syndrome, but habitually stress-dosing or from too high of a prescribed dose, can cause these symptoms and eventually the syndrome. Cushing's is also life-threatening, and causes a whole new set of problems. You want to be aware of the signs of too much cortisol, so you can discuss either your dosage or your stress-dosing practices with your practitioner.

Signs and symptoms of too much cortisol include:
- Weight gain
- Hypertension (high blood pressure)
- Poor short-term memory

- Irritability
- Excessive hair growth in women
- Red, ruddy face
- Extra fat around face
- Round, or 'moon' face
- Fatigue
- Poor concentration
- Menstrual irregularity
- "Buffalo hump"

Less common:
- Insomnia
- Recurrent infections
- Thin skin
- Severe stretch marks
- Easy bruising
- Depression
- Weak bones
- Acne
- Male-pattern balding in women
- Hip and shoulder weakness
- Swelling of feet and legs
- Diabetes

It is important to note that not all symptoms will be experienced.

If you notice these symptoms and they are increasing, it is important to discuss this with your endocrinologist. Be prepared to take with you a list of you dosage amounts and times – both regular and stress. A two-week period would be a good diary to take.

Any unusual symptoms should be discussed with your doctor or practitioner. Whether they are digestive related, menstrual, emotional, or any other type of symptoms. All physiological processes are affected by our hormonal system, and if you are adrenally insufficient, a whole domino-effect can take place when something is awry. Talk to your doctor, as it could be as simple as a change in dosage, or even lifesaving.

Because illness or injury can be life-threatening for persons with Adrenal Insufficiency, it is important to wear a medical identification bracelet or necklace so emergency personnel know you need special treatment. Again, *sudden stopping of steroids can lead to a life threatening Adrenal Crisis.*

Sources used in this chapter:

Stress Dosing – Oral and Injection, University of Kansas Medical Center

Managing Adrenal Insufficiency, NIG Clinical Center Patient Education Materials

Cushing's Syndrome and Disease Symptoms, The Pituitary Society

Chapter Five

Helping Family and Companions Understand

When you are diagnosed with a serious, chronic, and life-threatening illness, your family members can react in many different ways. This means you have lots of emotions to deal with in addition to your own.

Your family members will go through feelings of anger, disbelief, or even rejection. Many of these emotions will phase into understanding, while many of them will not only be permanent, but may even progress into harsher feelings. Almost every AI patient I've known has at least one family member who does not believe them, or does not understand the seriousness of the illness. Fortunately, many also have family members that become their lifeline and caregiver, as well. Unfortunately, while you, the patient, are the sick one and dealing with many emotions, new information, and starting treatment yourself, you also have to inform and educate your family. There are also the cases of new parents who have a baby born with CAH, and have to explain the illness, the extra care and concern that will be required regarding the child, make sure you have babysitters and caregivers who will not ignore signs of needing updosing, or worse yet, forget medication times, but .... there is a gene mutation that other family members may have.

The best scenario is that you have a close family member who has been concerned during the decline of health and realization of symptoms, doctors visits and testing, and diagnosis. Or, a portion of those. These family members, be it a spouse, sibling, child or other, can help relieve the load of not only notifying family, but helping them understand and assisting in education so they can be advocates and caregivers as well. This also helps relieve you of extra stress you obviously don't need as someone who does not make proper stress hormones.

If your endocrinologist has an assistant or patient education staff member, they can oftentimes make an appointment for the family to come in and participate in a presentation, discuss concerns, and ask questions. Other options are to show your family videos, or print out or order educational materials for the family to learn about your illness so they can look out for your needs. They could even read this book.

It is important for your family, before anybody else, understand your illness, not just because it is best for family to know anything first, but because those that are close to you need to know signs, symptoms, and procedures to help you if you are needing to stress dose, emergency inject, or if you are having an adrenal crisis. Family or those close to you can save your life – they can help you stress dose so your body does not begin the shutting down process, they can inject you with emergency meds so you do not have an adrenal crisis, faint and go into a coma with nobody knowing, and they can call doctors and emergency personnel on your behalf when you are unable to. They can stay with you until you get to a doctor, and until you are on the road to recovery. They can also answer questions about your recent health, behavior, symptoms, etc. It is sometimes impossible for the patient to do these things, because cognitive abilities are lessened and the person may not even be able to know the names of people to call, or even what to tell them is wrong, should they be able to. And if they faint or collapse, it can be too late. A member of my own support group passed away several months back because they were alone when they had an adrenal crisis.

When telling your family about your illness, it is not only important to give them educational handouts, but explain to them the seriousness of it! It is imperative that they know to watch for low cortisol signs, watch for illness, and watch the weather if you're salt wasting. If they cook for you and you are salt wasting, they need to know to provide salty foods or Himalayan pink salt for you to use (in case another family member needs to restrict their salt intake). They need to understand that brainfog, confusion, irritability, and a complete lack of comprehension are signs of you needing immediate help with stress dosing, an emergency injection, or calling your doctor. They need to recognize that if you seem to have respiratory illness, the flu, vomiting, diarrhea, etc., that you get stress dosing and they call the doctor on your behalf if you don't get better in 3 days. And most of all, they need to know *where* all of your medications are –particularly your emergency injection- *how* to give your emergency injection and when, and where your emergency letters are to give to paramedics or emergency personnel. They need to be able to articulate to such personnel the exact nature of your illness, what has been done before they got there or you arrived at the facility, and answer any questions on your behalf. It is best to have a trusted family member have a medical power of attorney, so they can act on your behalf if you are unconscious or in a coma. These actions on your behalf may easily save your life, or keep you from having permanent damage.

If you have family members who do not understand your illness, it is best to not try to 'make' them understand. Not only will it cause you extra stress and the need to stress dose and perhaps have an emergency, but they may resent your illness and your need for their services. They may come around in the future, but don't focus on convincing them that you are sick, or what to do. It would be terrible to force them to listen to instructions, and then find yourself unconscious or in a coma, and these people you've thought you could rely on do not know how to help you. It could cost your life. It is best to find a trusted family member and rely on that peace of mind.

That, or those, family members may need respite services. If you become ill and need them to attend to you for a long period of time, they may need some time away from having to worry about it and check on you. For this reason, it is important to have several family members or close friends aware of:
• what meds you need and when
• where your emergency meds are
• how to give emergency injections
• the exact nature of your illness
• what signs mean you need immediate assistance
• what procedures emergency personnel or surgical staff should be taking so they can advocate for you

Sources for educational materials to give your family members can be found in the "resources" chapter.

When a child is born with CAH, it can be a surprise, or it can be expected and prepared for. But it is still a shock, and can cause parents and grandparents to feel guilt. Since CAH requires both parents to carry the mutations, it is possible that one or both parents are either under treatment themselves, or are aware of somebody in their family who is – and will be familiar with signs, symptoms, medication needs, and other forms of care. If not, then the family needs to learn extremely quick! Infants require commencing treatment immediately, and infants and toddlers are not capable to inform the adults if signs and symptoms, so it is necessary that the adults around them are aware and always watching for them on their behalf.

Parents of a child with CAH also have to make decisions for their children that can be very difficult. Girls who are born with classic CAH at birth often have ambiguous genitals, and consideration must be made regarding corrective surgery such as what types and when. There are also decisions which need to be made regarding gender identity. Boys with classic CAH need to be monitored for TARTS (testicular adrenal rest tumors), fertility, as well as heart, blood pressure and other issues. Early puberty will also be a consideration. Organizations such as CARES can be extremely helpful with these issues, please see the resources section.

Chapter Six

Who Needs to Know

This is a tough issue. Some people are very private, while others wear their hearts on their sleeves. But when it comes to your life, these things must be put aside. Not only must we ensure that people are knowledgeable about precautions, emergency treatment, and the answers to questions that emergency personnel may have, but we must also be educators and teach people about the illness as they may be able to recognize symptoms in another person who is yet to be diagnosed – or another person who has been diagnosed, and needs emergency help.

The people you live with certainly must be extremely knowledgeable of all factors of your illness. They should know these basic things:

- Symptoms of the illness that may occur frequently and are uncomfortable, or need medication or treatment, special protocols, etc. to function normally.
- Signs of an impending crisis and how to help turn the situation around, or what to watch for that may indicate the situation getting worse.
- Signs of a current crisis
- Where emergency medications are
- How to give injections
  - What's been happening in your life recently so they can advise emergency personnel
  - All facts of your illness: what medications you take, what medications you have taken recently, who your doctor is, and where a copy of an emergency letter with instructions is kept

Other people who need to know as many of these details include (but are not limited to):

- Work supervisor
- Co-workers whom are close to you in proximity
- People you commute with
- People at your place of worship

•People at restaurants you may frequent
•Daycare providers
•Close neighbors

Basically, anybody who spends a lot of time with you, or is regularly around you, should be aware of as many of the above things so that they can recognize when you need help, and actually help you or get you immediate help. Friends and family who are willing to be trained in how to give emergency injections and what to tell emergency personnel are particularly valuable!

There are other 'people' who need to know. Your medical team is a good example. All doctors such as Primary Care physicians, specialists for other issues, dentists, etc. Their care is dependent on knowing your full picture, and they also need to know so that they do not do anything that may interfere with your treatment or exacerbate your illness. These physicians and providers can also watch for signs and symptoms you may not be as aware of and can communicate with you as well as your endocrinologist about these concerns. Pharmacists also need to know so that they can be sure and keep your medications on hand and realize the importance of timely refills or emergency refills. Also, make sure a copy of emergency orders from your endocrinologist is on file with any emergency room you may be taken to for treatment.

Your local Fire Department or Paramedic providers need to know your condition. You should make a point to visit with them and see that they have proper protocols in place for Adrenal Insufficiency patients, that they keep the proper medications such as Solu-Cortef on board, and if not- what their protocols are on using patients' own medications if they are called in an emergency. You can also file with them a copy of emergency instructions from your endocrinologist and any supporting documents. If the local fire department or paramedics are not knowledgeable regarding Adrenal Insufficiency and Adrenal Crisis, you can use this opportunity to educate them. There are many educational materials available from the resources listed in this book, and there are also petition templates that can be used to help you with an advocacy effort to get protocols changed.

You should always wear a medical alert bracelet. In the event you are in an accident or require medical assistance and are unable to speak for yourself, emergency personnel will be alerted to your condition and help you get the proper treatment as soon as possible. Bracelets are preferred, and most emergency responders look in that location. Try to get bracelets that are obviously 'medical' alerts, and aren't too ornamental and may look like just 'jewelry – they might get overlooked.

The bracelet can state several things, but most staff I've spoken with states that they prefer "Adrenal Insufficiency" or "Steroid Dependent" over "Addison's Disease" or "CAH", as most protocols are listed as AI. They not even be familiar that Addison's and CAH are, in fact, Adrenal Insufficiency. If you have the type of bracelet that allows, it can also have your endocrinologist's contact information, instructions on dosage required, or other emergency information. Some people use services that allow the personnel to log in or look online for further instructions using a special ID number. Staff have told me, however, that these take too much time and they don't usually have the time to get on a phone or tablet, find a website, and log in.

Chapter Seven

911 – EMERGENCY
ADRENAL CRISIS

An adrenal crisis is a true life or death situation. Without intervention, it can result in coma, organ failure, brain damage, or even death. These things can happen very quickly, and intervention is suggested within 45 to 60 minutes, preferably faster to avoid organ damage. If you think you are going into Adrenal Crisis, INJECT WITH YOUR SOLU-CORTEF or other steroid injection, and CALL 911.

What is Adrenal Crisis?

A very sudden, or abnormal worsening of adrenal insufficiency symptoms is called "Adrenal Crisis." If the patient has Addison's Disease, it is sometimes termed "Addisonian Crisis."

In many cases, the symptoms start worsening over a few days, sometimes a week, or at least in enough time that the person can updose or stress dose, or seek appropriate medical treatment before an actual Adrenal Crisis occurs. Unfortunately, a crisis can often come on without warning due to:
• an unknown infection or other bodily stressor
• an injury or an accident
• due to traumatic news or emotional situation

Sometimes, the Adrenal Crisis is the first indication of Addison's and leads the patient to diagnosis. In some cases, the patient passes away from the crisis, and the cause is not discovered until autopsy, as they were never diagnosed.

People who suffer from Adrenal Insufficiency who have weakness, nausea or vomiting need immediate emergency treatment to prevent an adrenal crisis and possible death. Injections of glucocorticoid hormones can save a person's life – common injections that are prescribed are:
•Solu-cortef (hydrocortisone)
•Dexamethasone
•Betamethasone

Symptoms of Adrenal Crisis

The symptoms of Adrenal Crisis are listed elsewhere in this book, and are many. Each person usually has a pattern, but even then, a surprise crisis can occur that has a completeky different set of symptoms! They can include the following, although not all symptoms will occur and there may be additional ones:

- Sudden, severe pain in the lower back, abdomen, or legs
- Severe vomiting and diarrhea
- Dehydration
- Low blood pressure
- Confusion and disorientation
- Mood alteration
- Headache/dizziness
- Lethargy
- Neurological dysfunction
- Pale skin/shivering/goosebumps
- Loss of consciousness

LACK OF IMMEDIATE TREATMENT OR MEDICAL INTERVENTION CAN LEAD TO COMA OR DEATH

Resources for this chapter:
National Health Institute
Adrenal Insufficiency United

ADRENAL INSUFFICIENCY
by: Professor Peter Hindmarsh

ADRENAL CRISIS - PATHWAY OF EVENTS

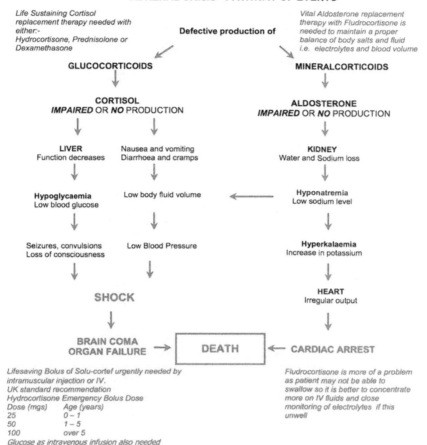

Life Sustaining Cortisol replacement therapy needed with either:- Hydrocortisone, Prednisolone or Dexamethasone

Defective production of

Vital Aldosterone replacement therapy with Fludrocortisone is needed to maintain a proper balance of body salts and fluid i.e. electrolytes and blood volume

GLUCOCORTICOIDS

MINERALCORTICOIDS

CORTISOL
***IMPAIRED* OR *NO* PRODUCTION**

ALDOSTERONE
***IMPAIRED* OR *NO* PRODUCTION**

LIVER
Function decreases

Nausea and vomiting
Diarrhoea and cramps

KIDNEY
Water and Sodium loss

Hypoglycaemia
Low blood glucose

Low body fluid volume

Hyponatremia
Low sodium level

Seizures, convulsions
Loss of consciousness

Low Blood Pressure

Hyperkalaemia
Increase in potassium

SHOCK

HEART
Irregular output

**BRAIN COMA
ORGAN FAILURE** → **DEATH** ← **CARDIAC ARREST**

Lifesaving Bolus of Solu-cortef urgently needed by intramuscular injection or IV.
UK standard recommendation
Hydrocortisone Emergency Bolus Dose

Dose (mgs)	Age (years)
25	0 – 1
50	1 – 5
100	over 5

Glucose as intravenous infusion also needed

Fludrocortisone is more of a problem as patient may not be able to swallow so it is better to concentrate more on IV fluids and close monitoring of electrolytes if this unwell

Reproduced from *Congenital Adrenal Hyperplasia: a comprehensive review* by Kathy Geertsma and Peter Hindmarsh with kind thanks to Elsevier Publishing

PART II - Daily Care

The remainder of this book deals with alternative methods of managing symptoms. It in no way implies that it can solely treat Adrenal Insufficiency or that you can stop taking your prescribed glucocorticoids and mineralocorticoids. It is simply an alternative outlook at managing symptoms and helping your body work *with* medications instead of fighting your body so it requires *more* medication. The point of this protocol is to support not only the adrenal glands themselves and their physiological processes, but to support other bodily functions dependent on adrenal response, and to make the quality of life increase for the better.

Holistic, complementary and alternative health methods are necessary to consistently follow for at least 4 weeks before any consideration of change, elimination of components, is discussed. Addressing the root of any problem is not as hastily responsive to a synthetic 'pill' that addresses a symptom. If you are not willing to be compliant or not give this lifestyle change a chance, just remember that even orthodox, allopathic medicine treatments can often take months, as in radiation, chemotherapy, etc. We are talking about your wellness and quality of life, and patience is a virtue! If you are a 'give me a pill and I'll feel better' mentality for all of the symptoms and things that go along with Adrenal Insufficiency, you should investigate holistic methods a bit more before beginning this lifestyle. Just keep your eyes on the prize – a better quality of life!

This lifestyle and mindset change involves *Daily Care*, the subject of the remainder of the book.

Chapter Eight

Daily Care
Awareness

With Adrenal Insufficiency, circumstances start a chain reaction by putting stress on your body. Fighting a cold, even if you're successful in warding it off, can use up available cortisol and require up dosing. A change in weather resulting in high humidity and hot temperature can cause dehydration in salt wasters. If you're diabetic and you've been overdoing the carbs and sugars causing the need for more insulin, that can put stress on your body and use up cortisol, as well. A birthday party you've woken up early to prepare for, for example. The list goes on and on.

Be aware of your surroundings every day, and even a day or two in advance. Make sure you are preparing yourself using techniques such as diet, water, supplements, activities, and other modalities. For example, if you know the weather is changing to become very hot and humid, start as soon as possible in consuming enough water, eating salt, and watching the amount of potassium-containing foods or supplements you're consuming. Make arrangements to do indoor activities, or if outdoor activities are necessary, plan them early in the morning, or early evening.

The following things are those which should be monitored. The first list is things which should be monitored once, or several times a day until you establish a pattern you are familiar with. This is especially important because not everybody's symptoms are the same, or are 'textbook.' Keep a record in a journal of the following for at least 10-14 days:

•**Blood pressure**. Check BP while lying down when you wake, take again when standing up. Also check your blood pressure at least 2 more times per day first lying down for at least 3 minutes, and then after standing. Also check and record if any unusual circumstances arise, such as strenuous activity, a dizzy spell, bad news, etc. It will help you learn your body's reaction to such things.

•**Pulse**. Your pulse is checked at the same time, and should be recorded as well. Pulse can be checked any other time, and it is a good and inexpensive idea to carry a finger pulse meter. They also check oxygen.

•**Blood Sugar**. Blood sugar often lowers and rises along with cortisol, and you can learn how your blood sugar might be an indicator useful to you. If you start feeling out of sorts and a pattern develops that your blood sugar is lower at those times, then this can be a good indicator in the future and a way to check if perhaps your cortisol is indeed low.

•**Journal how you're feeling**.

Pain level – make yourself a scale of 1-10, and make any note of specifics. Some people notice they get flank pain, or leg pain, if cortisol starts getting low. Or they start getting headaches and muscle twitches if getting dehydrated. If you see that these things occur along with other signs, you'll know in the future how to start gauging symptoms. Perhaps you get twitches and headaches at the same time that your blood pressure drops. This is a good indicator of dehydration and the need for sodium. Other patterns may develop.

Emotionally – some people experience moodiness, tearfulness, anxiety, etc. when cortisol is low, but also experience agitation and hyperactivity if cortisol is high. These patterns will start to make sense with other patterns during this monitoring time.

Cognitively – many people experience cognitive dysfunction, ranging from 'brain fog' to complete lack of comprehension. Sometimes people are described as 'spacy,' 'somewhere else', or even 'stroke-like.'

Appetite – while there is no norm or rule to how this manifests, each person has his or her own indicators. Some patients report lack of appetite and feeing nauseated, others become hungrier than usual, and some notice no changes in appetite. Salt wasters will notice a craving for salty foods, such as pickles, etc. This can be a big indicator for the need of sodium, especially if blood pressure is dropping and other indicators you have noticed in your pattern.

List of meds and supplements – notice if you feel better with certain supplements, or worse with others. If you are taking them only a few days a week and you feel better when taking them, perhaps you need to discuss with your practitioner the possibility of taking them more frequently. If they are making you feel worse, perhaps your body is not absorbing them properly, there is a contraindication with another supplement or med, etc. Never add a supplement to your routine without discussing with a practitioner who would have a better idea of contraindications, conversion factors that may be affected by other supplements and medications, etc.

Diet for the day – Keep track of what you eat and when you eat it while doing this journaling. If certain foods are causing you problems, it will be worth investing time or consultation with a practitioner to see what the nutrients in the food are and how they may be reacting with your meds or supplements, etc. For example, if your blood pressure has gone up significantly and consistently and you are a salt waster on Fludrocortisone, you also take supplemental electrolytes, and you are eating a large quantity of foods with sodium, you can see where this may need some adjustment. There can also be issues with foods with potassium, foods that lower cortisol, etc.

The following things should be thought about several days in advance:

•**Weather** – Keep an eye on heat, heat index, humidity, storms, etc. If you are salt wasting, you will find that these changes can contribute to dehydration, can cause bloating, and other factors. It is good to know a few days in advance if this type of weather is advancing, so you can hydrate with water and electrolytes, or up your sodium and fludrocortisone (if your practitioner has advised you to make necessary changes with your fludro).

•**Menus** – Make sure you are eating a balanced diet each day – proper sodium, not too many foods that lower cortisol, and general good eating (discussed elsewhere in this book), and perhaps increasing sodium and other nutrients as needed due to weather and activities coming up. Make sure you have enough water on hand.

•**Activities** – Make sure you are not overdoing your schedule. Always leave 'me' time in each day, and schedule it in your diary or planner like any other appointment, and do not cancel it! Try not to schedule too many activities too many days in a row, and also pay attention to weather. If it is going to be 109 with 85%

humidity, it is probably not a good idea to schedule outdoor activities if you are a salt waster, for example!

Each individual day you should consider how you feel based on the patterns and signs you established in the record-keeping, and with the knowledge you have established a couple of days earlier, it is then possible to plan your day in a way that will help your body not fight itself and possibly avoid a downward spiral from starting or avoid a potential crisis.

It is possible you may have to alter your menu for the day. For example, if your blood pressure is at a low and you are dizzy, you then know you need to add more salt, and avoid being in the heat. If you feel your blood sugar is getting low, you may need to change your meal times and add more protein to that particular meal.

Chapter Nine

Daily Care
Diet

Most people understand that 'diet' doesn't mean an eating plan for maintaining weight, but rather, an eating plan to maintain good health. Diet requirements are different for each individual, based on their own chemical makeup and illnesses. Not every person who has Adrenal Insufficiency will find that everything in the following plan is adequate for their management, depending on what other illnesses may co-exist with their AI. Generally, however, this is a good rule of thumb for AI.

Following is my recommended protocol for general healthy eating. However, each person's chemistry and medical conditions call for modifications. For example, a person with Hashimotos (hypothyroid) would not eat as many portions of cruciferous vegetables. Following this protocol are the adrenal specific modifications. This way, you have good guidelines for the healthy members of your family, and modifications for your eating, as well.

Start Your Day Right

It is very important to eat protein within 15-20 minutes of rising, in order to raise glucagons and help blood sugar and insulin work properly throughout the day. Blood sugar and cortisol are very connected, so in addition to controlling blood sugar and hypoglycemic episodes during the day, this is important for those with AI. Cheese, a piece of turkey bacon, yogurt (especially with active enzymes!), a few nuts, are all good choices. This is a very important way to start your day, as it sets up your body to work properly when all of your other methods are made.

It is also very important to eat regular meals at consistent times ... 3 times a day, with a snack mid-morning and mid-afternoon. This will keep the blood sugar level, and will also help the circadian rhythm in order for the purposes of energy, sleep and endocrine functions/hormone production. Watch your portions – a portion of anything should be about the size of a deck of cards, or fit in the palm of your hand.

Refined Foods

Avoid sugars. For a sweetener, use stevia. Avoid processed foods ... prepackaged and box mixes. They are FULL of things you don't need, and missing many of the things you *do* need. If not using fresh vegetables, do not used can, but use frozen. They retain the enzymes needed by the body as well as a large amount of the nutrients. Steaming vegetables, whether fresh or frozen, also helps retain the nutrients. Do not BOIL or cook vegetables in water. Light stir-fry with a dash of olive oil and some Braggs Aminos (sold in a bottle like soy sauce) and stir-fry them with any seasoning you want (as long as it's not a blend that has added sugars). Avoid cooking with any oils other than olive or coconut. It is ok to use butter, but in very limited amounts – just to add taste to something!

Refined carbohydrates have a devastating affect on health, particularly for pre- and current diabetics, as carbohydrates turn to sugar in the body. . Refining grains strips out most minerals, oils, and fiber necessary for the optimal functioning of our minds and bodies. After years of eating noodles, refined cereals, pancakes and waffles, cookies, etc. subtle mineral and vitamin deficiencies can develop that sooner or later manifest as chronic ailments and disease. When laboratory tests start showing deficiencies, the problem is already manifesting. Stripping the germ and bran fro a kernel of wheat, for example, removes a significant portion of its vitamins: B-1, B-2, B-3, B-5, B-6, biotin, folic acid, as well as chromium, iron, calcium, potassium, magnesium, and more. A good example is the fact that in white bread, the loss of nutrients from refining is very high .... A 96% loss in vitamin E alone, for example.

Some suggestions for replacements can be:

Pasta: Spaghetti Squash, Shiritaki Noodles, or whole grain pasta
Sugar: Stevia, honey, agave
Flours: In cooking, use coconut flours. Try using flourless recipes. Avoid foods that are breaded or have unnecessary flours. For thickeners, use instead Greek yogurt, coconut flour or pureed pumpkin.

Breads: Use sprout breads (such as Ezekiel bread, or make your own), as well as "Flat-outs", and "Fold-its".

Other carbohydrates: These food items can also replace these refined foods in order to obtain your complex carbohydrates. Corn, brown or wild rice, millet, amaranth, quinoa, and spelt are good choices. Another way to obtain your Complex Carbohydrates is with winter squash (butternut, acorn, blue hubbard, etc.), sweet potatoes and yams.

Eat Your Veggies

Vegetables add numerable vitamins, minerals, enzymes and fiber to the diet as well as work in combination with other foods to provide absorption of necessary nutrients from the diet as a whole. A significant amount of fiber is contained in vegetables. If cooking these vegetables, do *not* boil in water. Most, if not all, of the nutrients are cooked out, and the enzymes are destroyed. Raw is best, and next best is steaming. When steaming, be sure you use a lid and you can add flavors to the water to permeate the vegetables such as juice of a lemon, garlic, etc. Potatoes should be limited, as they are extremely starchy and full of carbohydrates. Good replacements are turnips, cauliflower and water chestnuts. Instead of fried potatoes, try frying some sliced water chestnuts in a sparse amount of olive oil. For 'mashed,' try mashing steamed cauliflower or turnips with Greek yogurt instead of butter. Instead of chips, try pork rinds or make kale or radish trips in the oven by thin slicing radishes (or cut up kales), spraying with olive oil and roasting in the oven. A "Misto" makes it very affordable to use the correct amounts of spray and not using propellants like in canned oil sprays. It is a great investment! There are really lots of options with vegetables; using spices, you can change them up in many different ways. For instance, with green beans, you can steam them with onions, or with garlic and lemon, or with curry powder, etc. It's all dependent on your taste. Spices are a great, calorie-free way to change flavors on repetitive foods. It is important not to eat canned vegetables. The nutrients have all been diminished, and all enzymes have been stripped from commercially canned vegetables. If vegetables are used in a salad, please do not use anymore than 2 TBS of a salad dressing, preferably using low fat dressings. Balsamic vinegar and oil dressings are good to use, or spray your salad with olive oil from your Misto, and season with your favorite seasonings.

Proteins

Use proteins from 'whole' sources, and cut back on processed meats. You should have at least 2 servings per day. Your two servings of protein can be made up of Fish, Fowl, Eggs and Meat as well as Legumes (beans, split peas, lentils, etc.), Milk products (yogurt, cottage cheese, cheese, etc.) and Seeds/Nuts/Nut Butters. The latter should be used sparingly as they are very high in fat. However, each seed or nut can be targeted for certain needs. For example, Brazil nuts are good for lowering cholesterol if eaten in moderation. When choosing meat, opt for organic whenever possible. They contain fewer antibiotics and have more nutritional value. Buy fresh, and freeze portions yourself. Although it is important to eliminate excess fat from the diet, you should always buy red meat that has 'marbled' fat running throughout it. This fat is natural to the meat, and is a balanced portion. Fat is necessary for health and digestion, but not excess fat. Marbled fat contained within meat naturally is not 'excess' fat." However, the hard 'rind' fat on meat should be cut off. Broiling is an ideal way to prepare your meat products, or using a George Foreman-type grill. Both let excess fat drain, are fast, and have easy cleanup. Never add oils or fats to a cooking vessel when preparing meat – the meat has just enough fat already contained in it. Only add oil or fat if it is needed to prevent sticking. A small amount of olive oil from a Misto, or coconut oil, is ideal. Never eat the same protein for more than 1 serving per day (Example: Fish at lunch, beef at dinner. Or chicken at lunch and fish at dinner, etc.)

Fruits

Make sure you have raw fruits in your daily diet; one serving with each meal. The amount should be more in warmer months and less in cooler notes. Fruits can be added to salads, or used as a snack in the afternoon along with a protein (example: sliced apples and cheese). Fruit salad is a good choice for a desert, such as a combination of peaches, strawberries, blueberries and raspberries. Always wash them thoroughly, and sprinkle stevia on them if needed. Fruits are high in all nutrients and are strong antioxidants.

If you are diabetic, you will want to look at the glycemic level of each fruit before placing it in your menu.

Fermented Foods

Be sure you have one serving per day of fermented foods to maintain a good bacteria level and a healthy intestinal flora. The choices would include yogurts with active enzymes (very important that it is marked with active enzymes), unpasteurized miso, Tempeh, or kefir. Even a small shot of Apple Cider Vinegar. This is a very important part of the daily diet.

Juicing

Juicing is a helpful method for body healing and achieving homeostasis. Juicing is not merely the 'juice' of certain foods, but utilizing the entire food, and manually starting the digestive enzyme process while preserving all enzymes. When using just the 'juice' of a food, the enzymes are not present, and the digestive process has not started. Juicing uses the whole food, provides all vitamins, minerals and enzymes of the food but in a liquid state that has started to digest when ingested.

Up to ninety percent of fiber is removed from the raw foods when juicing, while leaving all minerals, vitamins, enzymes, etc.

While preparing these juice meals, it is suggested to 'chew' something, whether it is mint gum or other. The chewing action starts the digestive process in the body (as does slow chewing when eating solid foods).

Juicing recipes that may be of help for your particular concerns are at the end of this chapter.

Never juice more than what can be consumed within an hour. When juicing the foods, you are activating the enzymes in the foods, which begin digestion. The food will start destroying itself after that time and will be of no value, and will become rancid soon. Never use canned juice in its place – it is not the same type of 'juice." Canned or prepared juices do not have the enzymes and the 'food' qualities of juicing, they are simply 'juice,' not a food.

Oils

Two tablespoons of Coconut Oil are recommended each day. Coconut oil is not metabolized the same as other oils, and will fulfill the need for oils in the body and intestinal tract, while helping with weight issues the client has expressed concern about. The benefits of coconut oil are numerous. If you have a sweet tooth and love chocolate, you can get both your chocolate fix and your coconut oil in one fell swoop by making "Chocolate Delight." Melt 2 TBS of coconut oil in a small mixing container, add 2 TBS ditched cocoa and 1 TBS of stevia and stir well. Drop coarse sea salt on top. Freeze for at least 30 minutes, and then break into pieces and enjoy. You will notice no weight gain, acne or other symptoms commercial candy causes, and will be getting the health benefits of your coconut oil and even the benefits of chocolate (without the waxes, oils, sugars, etc.). If you ingest the full amount in one day, you may want to use sprayed coconut oil that day for any cooking.

Adrenal-specific Eating

The following foods should be avoided, or kept at a minimum, as they are known to lower cortisol:

Dark chocolate
Microgreens (under 14 days old, due to high levels of Vitamin C, known to lower cortisol)
Omega-3 fatty acids
Citrus fruits and other fruits high in Vitamin C
Beans and Barley
Whey protein
Eggs
Brown rice
Wheat bread

If you have low aldosterone and are a salt-waster, the following foods should also be avoided:

Any diuretics:
Caffeine
Watermelon
Tomatoes
Cucumber
Cranberry Juice
Carrot
Eggplant
Artichoke

Celery
Grapes
Asparagus
Bananas (high in potassium)
   Coconut water (although it is high in sodium and other electrolytes, it is extremely high in potassium)
   Sports Drinks (PowerAde, Gator-Ade, etc.) (These drinks are formulated for athletes and endurance sports, and are extremely high in carbohydrates as such. They are formulated for an athlete to ingest during training and competition when carbs are used up immediately)
   Coconut Water (although praised for it's high content of electrolytes, there is a high potassium content and a relatively low sodium content; the opposite of what salt-wasters need.)

If you need to ingest any of the above salt-wasting foods due to other illnesses, etc., it is important to maintain a proper water/sodium/potassium balance by adding additional water and electrolytes.

Fats and Proteins

Fats should be mostly saturated and monounsaturated from natural foods.

Polyunsaturated fats should be kept low, as these increase free radical damage (accelerating aging), negatively affect thyroid signaling, lower testosterone levels and increase estrogen levels. This fat can come from meats such as beef and lamb, butter, eggs, coconut oil, olive oil, macadamia nuts, etc. If you choose to keep your fats low, just be sure you cook in healthy natural fats such as coconut oil, add olive oil to salads and base your meals around protein sources such as beef and eggs that contain fat and cholesterol. Adequate protein is critical to adrenal function, but eating more than you need is not helpful.

People with AI have low levels of cortisol and increased levels of catecholamines, including norepinephrine. Diets with too much protein tend to make people with AI feel nervous, anxious and 'jittery,' and make them prone to 'crashing,' or having cortisol lows thus being at risk for adrenal crisis. These high protein levels are often made obvious to the individual through excessive body odor (more of a body odor than a yeast odor), and are a signal for the individual to reduce their protein intake. Moderate protein diets also provide a moderate amount of tyrosine, which is also a dopamine precursor – an important neurotransmitter that increases energy, while too much tyrosine makes the imbalance between cortisol and catecholamines worse.

Likewise, a low protein diet causes the metabolism to slow down, as tyrosine is needed to form the thyroid hormone and high quality protein is needed to convert the thyroid hormone to its active form in the liver. It is a very fine line, as high protein diets slow down the metabolism, due to the amino acids cysteine and tryptophan are thyroid suppressive in high quantities.

Carbohydrates, Sugars and Calories

Although most people are worried about excess weight, those who take supplementary cortisol are extremely worried. Therefore, they stay shy of carbohydrates. However, a very low carbohydrate diet damages metabolism. Severely restricting carbs for long periods of time can cause AI in and of itself, and can also cause severe glucose deprivation which forces the adrenal glands into action to maintain blood sugar levels, a serious problem with any adrenal illness.

Many people with AI do well on a rough carbohydrate to protein ration of 2:1, along with good levels of natural fats (particularly well-marbled red meat). An effective carb count for AI is 75 to 100 grams.

By all means, avoid refined sugar! High sugar diets reduce insulin sensitivity, use up vital minerals such as magnesium, zinc, chromium and manganese and put a great deal of stress on the adrenal glands. It is important to limit natural sugars and sweet fruits, as well.

Both extremely low calorie diets and low carb diets (<75 grams) cause metabolic slowdown and will worsen symptoms of the adrenal illness. In the low energy situations created by long-term practice of such diets, the thyroid often deactivates itself by reversing the active hormone T3 into the inactive reverse T3 (rT3). When this happens, the order of the iodine atom ring reverses and creates a mirror image of T3. Reverse T3 is often not tested for by doctors but its symptoms are similar to those of primary hypothyroidism, i.e., low body temperature, dry skin, slow metabolism, fatigue, hair loss, sensitivity to cold, and many more. The AI itself is often a factor behind elevated rT3 levels and straightening out the AI often sorts this problem out. The last thing a person exhibiting rT3 elevation should do is to do an extreme diet for weight loss. You want to address the root problem, eat a healthy diet for the condition, and a good and proper weight will come. When high levels of reverse T3 are present, the body is in a state of perceived starvation from which even thyroid hormone will not help. Individuals should always be on a special diet for health, not weight!

Salt/Sodium

AI patients who suffer low levels of the hormone Aldosterone (salt wasters) need to pay particular attention to extra salt in the diet, as well as sodium in supplements. More information on this in the *Hydration* section.

Timing of Meals

Whatever you do, do *not* skip meals! The importance of eating regular meals cannot be underestimated. A breakfast, even small, with protein within 30 minutes of waking is extremely important to signal the production of glucagon, which will set up proper insulin balance throughout the day, and may prevent afternoon hypoglycemia episodes in the afternoons.

Three to four meals a day is imperative with AI. Going long periods without eating, or missing meals, stimulates an increase in adrenaline in order for the body to maintain blood sugar levels, which stresses the adrenal glands. You should not go for more than 5-6 hours without eating a meal; 3 meals a day eaten 5-6 hours apart, or 4 meals a day slightly more closely spaced, is an effective plan. By implementing this regimen, as well as eating meals at roughly the same time every day can help the circadian rhythm of cortisol and other important hormones react more appropriately.

Alcohol

Corticosteroids can irritate the stomach, and alcohol can compound this action. Avoid alcohol; it can also cause random blood pressure highs and lows.

Adrenal Specific Juicing
The following ingredients are particularly recommended for the AI patient. A couple of recipes follow the list.

Romaine Lettuce. Although a member of the lettuce family, Romaine Lettuce has an entirely different chemical composition from that of Head Lettuce (Iceberg). In Great Britain it is known as "Cos Lettuce." The juice of Romaine Lettuce, with the addition of a small amount of Kelp (seaweed) has been found to contain properties conducive to helping the activity of the Adrenal Cortex in its function of secreting hormones, and keeps the body in balance. Its particular value is in its rich sodium content, which is 60% higher than it's potassium content. This makes it one of the most beneficial juices for conditions affecting the Adrenal Glands. A person with Adrenal Insufficiency requires the maximum amount of vital organic sodium with a relatively low percentage of potassium to compensate for Adrenal hormone deficiency. This specifically proportioned juice is therefore essentially very relative to just such a person's needs.

Pomegranate. Pomegranate seeds are rich in lignans which provide anti-oxidant, anti-cancer and estrogenic properties. The pomegranate's phytoestrogenic properties are full of 17-alfa-estradiol, which is similar to estrogens produced in the female body. The properties in the pomegranate are SERMs – Selective Estrogen Receptor Modulators which is a compound that attaches itself to an estrogen receptor so there is no room for the antagonistic estrogen to attach itself to the cell, so it is also helpful to women who experience estrogen dominance and are prone to breast cancer, endometriosis, fibroids, PMS and thyroid nodules.

Beet. This is one of the most valuable juices for helping to build up the red corpuscles of the blood and tone up the blood generally. Women, particularly, have been benefited by drinking at least one pint of a combination of carrot and beet juice daily. The 20% potassium content furnishes the general nourishment for all the physiological functions of the body, while the 8% content of chlorine furnishes a splendid organic cleanser of the liver, kidneys, and gall bladder, also stimulating the activity of the lymph throughout the entire body. <u>WARNING</u>: Taken alone, beet juice, in greater quantities than a wineglass at a time, may cause a cleansing reaction that may make a person feel nauseated and/or dizzy. Thus, any juicing recipes that contain beet juice should be followed carefully.

Spinach. Spinach is the most vital food for the entire digestive tract, both the alimentary section of the body (the stomach, duodenum, and small intestines) and for the large intestine or colon, and it has been so recognized since time immemorial. In raw spinach, Nature has furnished man with the finest organic material for the cleansing, reconstruction, and regeneration of the intestinal tract. It is imperative after any cleanses, flushes, or diarrhea episodes, that the system be replaced by an organic alkaline solution such as raw fruit juices to prevent an inevitable water deficiency in the body. Also, if this replacement is not made, one runs the risk of repetition. Raw spinach juice effectively cleanses and helps to heal not only the lower bowels but also the entire intestinal tract. The spinach works by natural means to repair the most essential damage first; it is not always apparent to the individual where in the body the work if regeneration is progressing. Results may not be noticeable sometimes for as long as six weeks or two months after daily ingestion of this juice. (Spinach should never be eaten when cooked unless we are particularly anxious to accumulate oxalic acid crystals in the kidneys, with subsequent kidney problems and stones. When spinach is cooked or canned, the oxalic acid atoms become inorganic as a result of excessive heat and may form oxalic acid crystals in the kidneys.)

Carrot. Raw carrot juice may be taken indefinitely in any reasonable quantities. It has the effect of helping to normalize the entire system. It is the richest source of Vitamin A which the body can quickly assimilate and contains also an ample supply of Vitamins B, C, D, E, G, and K. It helps to promote the appetite and is an aid to digestion. It is a natural solvent for ulcerous and cancerous conditions, and is resistant to infections, doing most efficient work in conjunction with the adrenal glands. It helps prevent infections of the eyes and throat as well as the tonsils and sinuses and the respiratory organs generally. Intestinal and liver diseases are sometimes due to a lack of certain of the elements contained in properly prepared raw carrot juice. . Carrot juice is composed of a combination of elements, which nourish the entire system, helping to normalize its weight as well as its chemical balance. NOTE: Skin discoloration can be observed with the use of carrot juice INTERESTING FACT: By means of the latest super-microscopes, it has been possible to determine that the carrot juice molecule is exactly analogous to that of the blood molecule, a most interesting and revealing fact.

RECIPES:

Adrenal Elixir One
16 oz. beet and beet tops
Scoop of seaweed powder

Adrenal Elixir Two
16 oz. Romaine lettuce
Scoop of seaweed powder

Adrenal Elixir Three
16 oz. Pomegranate
Scoop of seaweed powder

Adrenal Elixir Four
7 oz. carrot
5 oz. Romaine lettuce
4 oz. Pomegranate
Scoop of seaweed powder

Adrenal Elixir Five
7 oz. Celery
5 oz. Romaine lettuce
4 oz. Spinach leaves and stems
Scoop of seaweed powder

• • •

*If other juicing recipes are enjoyed, add 1 scoop of kelp to each recipe
for minerals and electrolytes/sodium.*

Chapter Ten

Daily Care
Hydration

During the heat, when you're exercising, etc., people will say, "Drink plenty of water!" or, "Stay hydrated!" Is there a difference between the two? The answer is a resounding "Yes!"

Although life is not possible without water and the human body is made up of 80% water, there *is* such a thing as 'too much of a good thing.' Without a proper balance of electrolytes, particularly sodium, you can develop water intoxication, or hyponatremia, which means too much water and not enough sodium. That can cause your blood pressure to drop to coma levels and immediate intervention (very similar to an adrenal crisis, and can certainly quickly lead to a low-cortisol induced adrenal crisis).

One of sodium's jobs is to balance the fluids in and around your cells. Drinking too much water causes an imbalance, and the liquid moves from your blood to inside your cells, making them swell. If the swelling were to be inside the brain, it requires immediate treatment.

This explains how people can drink plenty of water, become bloated, and still be dehydrated – not enough electrolytes.

Infants, children, elderly and those with chronic illnesses (especially ones affecting endocrine and blood pressure issues) are particularly prone to water intoxication. This is one of the reasons many pediatricians advise infants to deink only breast milk or formula, because their systems are not yet ready for large amounts of water. There have been deaths from hazing rituals, and coaches requiring students to drink lots of water.

Salt is just as important to the body as water. It plays a major role in health, and feeds nutritional mineral elements to our cells, sanitizes and cleanses toxic waste from our system, and keeps water levels properly maintained in the body. It also is responsible for the balance of acids and bases in the body, and provides the movement of electrical currents to all muscles and cells. Without the proper electrical current, you will have trouble with muscles, nerves, cells operating correctly, and many other issues. Stress or infection demand an extra supply of salt, and out salt reserves can be depleted when sick or injured, or even over-stressed.

In nature, sodium chloride (salt) never occurs in pure form. A multitude of essential major and trace elements are in its crystals. Here is a partial list of these minerals and their function in human metabolism:

Sodium – Essential to digestion and metabolism, regulates body fluids, nerve and muscular functions.

Chlorine – Essential component of body fluids.

Calcium – Needed for bone mineralization.

Magnesium – Dissipates sodium excess, forms and hardens bones, ensures mental development and sharpens intelligence, promotes assimilation of carbohydrates, assures metabolism of Vitamin C and Calcium, retards the aging process and dissolves kidney stones.

Sulfur – Controls energy transfer in tissue, bone and cartilage cells, essential for protein compounds.

Silicon – Needed in carbon metabolism and for skin and hair balance.

Iodine – Vital for energy production and mental development, ensures production of thyroid hormones, needed for auto-defense mechanism (lymphatic system).

Bromine – In magnesium bromide form, a nervous system regulator and restorer, vital for pituitary hormonal function.

Phosphorous – Essential for biochemical synthesis and nerve cell functions related to the brain, constituent of phosphoproteins, nucleoproteins and phospholipids.

Vanadium – Of greater value for tooth bone calcification than fluorine, tones cardiac and nervous systems, reduces cholesterol, regulates phospholipids in blood, a catalyst for oxidation of many biological substances.

Electrolytes are minerals in your blood and other body fluids that carry an electrical charge. Some are positives, some are negatives, and both are needed to not only carry the electrical charges, but to move water and fluids through the cells, and not just have them sit and make you bloated and not reach the cells that need them. This is called 'Third Spacing' and you can actually become dehydrated, even though your body is full of fluids.

Electrolytes affect the amount of water in your body, the acidity of your blood, your muscle function, and other important processes. You lose electrolytes when you sweat, and you must replace them by drinking fluids that contain electrolytes. Water does not contain electrolytes.

Common electrolytes include:
Calcium, Chloride, Magnesium, Phosphorous, Potassium and Sodium.

Electrolytes can be acids, bases and salts. Not all 'salts' are sodium.

Symptoms of water intoxication are very similar to a heatstroke, and include being hot, having a headache, nausea and diarrhea. If you don't get help right away, the condition can quickly lead to swelling in the brain, seizures and coma. Get to the emergency room as soon as possible, where doctors can inject concentrated salt water to ease swelling and reverse the problems.

If you plan on drinking large amounts of water, make sure you have enough sodium, and/or electrolytes. Be cautious with many commercial waters that state they are fortified with electrolytes. Some do not include sodium, the *one* electrolyte that is necessary to balance the water! Be sure you look for sodium. Electrolytes are available in numerous commercial tablets, powders and drops. You can find them at many grocers, drug stores, health food stores and naturopathic/chiropractic clinics. Use them once a day, but you'll know if you've overdone it ...you will probably get diarrhea, and your blood pressure could increase. If you are in the heat and drinking lots of water and begin to feel sick and dizzy, you probably need electrolytes.

Those with heart issues that stem from the Renin-Angiotensin system, or adrenal issues with low aldosterone need to be particularly careful with balancing salt and water, as Aldosterone is the hormone in the body that balances the distribution of both and maintains the proper balance, with or without heat or exhaustion, but on a minute-by-minute basis.

What types of salt are recommended? Himalayan Pink, Fleur de Sel, Celtic and Grey Sea Salt. In case of sudden symptoms of salt depletion, pickle juice is a good fast drink.

What forms of electrolytes are recommended? Powders, tablets (some are flavored!) and drops. In case of electrolyte deficiency and sudden onset of symptoms, one of the best remedies is Marine Plasma, and emergency electrolyte packets made for camping and first aid kits.

If you are having electrolyte deficiency issues, be careful with teas and foods that are diuretics. Diuretics cause you to lose lots of fluids through urination. These include caffeinated drinks, watermelon, celery and many other foods. If you take a prescription diuretic due to Congestive Heart Failure or other illness, please make sure you have adequate electrolytes.

A good supplement you can make at home is called *Sole* (pronounced SO-lay, as in 'sun'). Sole is an age-old form of Brine Water, useful for not only dehydration and salt-wasting illnesses, but for supplementation for many other issues.

Sole is known to help balance the pH factor of your body, and is also a known detox to rid the body of heavy metals such as lead, mercury, arsenic, amalgam and calcium. It does this by breaking up their molecular structures. By breaking up these structures, your body is able to metabolize them so that the body can then eliminate them. Even animal proteins, oftentimes difficult to break down and eliminate, is said to be flushed by the urine through using Sole.

But detoxing and elimination is not the only thing wonderful about Sole. The concentrated solution can supply the body with the 84 minerals found in its base, Himalayan Pink Salt. This is extremely helpful and useful for hydration, and for those who suffer salt wasting, or who work in the heat, or are athletic. It is also known to help normalize blood pressure. Research also shows that its regular use can help dissolve and eliminate sediments that lead to stones and various forms of rheumatism like arthritis and kidney and gallstones. Another great benefit is the ability to help with skin diseases by cleaning from inside out.

One teaspoon of sole not only contains a concentration of all 84 minerals found in Himalayan Salt, but 478 mg of Sodium.

Below is a list of benefits that have shown to be enjoyed by using Sole:

•Using a combination of Pink Himalayan Salt and water, as in Sole, blood pressure regulation has been achieved.

•Sole has been shown to be vital in balancing the sugar levels in the blood.

•Sole is important for the generation of hydroelectric energy in your body's cells.

•Sole is vital to the nerve cells for communication of electrical impulses and information processes.

•Sole has been shown to be important in the absorption of food particles through the intestinal tract.

•Sole has been shown to clear congestion of the sinuses.

•Sole improves circulation.

•Sole is believed to be essential for the prevention of muscle cramps.

Sole can be made easily at home. Below is a recipe and instructions for using it. And remember, any nutrient to help repair damage to your body can take time for results to be evident. Sometimes 2 to 4 weeks, sometimes up to 4 months. And, as the body uses nutrients on a daily basis, it is important to be extremely consistent in their usage. Consistency with a product like Sole is particularly important if you have electrolyte problems, hydration issues and a salt-wasting illness.

SOLE RECIPE

Use large Pink Himalayan Salt stones or chunks (you can purchase them specifically for making Sole from some retailers)

Step 1: Remember that if you keep adding salt to a glass of water, it will get to a point where the water becomes saturated. You will know this has happened when the salt sits at the bottom of the container and does not dissolve. This is what we are striving for! Place 1 inch of Himalayan salt in a glass jar. Add 2 to 3 inches of spring water above the stones, completely covering them and let sit overnight.

Step 2: If all of the salt has dissolved, add some more to the water. The Sole is ready when you add salt that does not dissolve anymore. As you use up the Sole, you can keep adding more water and more salt until it is again saturated. There should always be undissolved salt at the bottom of the container, so that you are sure the water is 'saturated.'

Recommended Usage: Each morning before eating or drinking anything, add one teaspoon of Sole to a glass of Spring water and drink (unless your practitioner suggests otherwise). Keep the container covered with a lid so it does not evaporate. It will NOT go bad.... Salt is a natural anti-bacterial and fungicide, so it will not spoil, and does not need to be refrigerated).

Chapter Eleven

Daily Care
Supplements

Supplements are very misunderstood. People often call any 'supplement' a 'vitamin,' even if it's a mineral. Supplements are over-the-counter formulations that 'supplement' something you're not getting enough of. Some supplements are over-the-counter in the US, but are only by prescription in other countries, such as DHEA. Therefore, it doesn't make sense to 'poo-poo' a supplement, when in another country it just might be a pharmaceutical prescription! Also, many prescriptions are supplements. Prescription Vitamin D3, for example, or even hydrocortisone or cortisol (corticosteroid, or glucocorticoid). Hydrocortisone is not a medical treatment that causes an action, but rather a supplemental amount of cortisol that is needed because you do not make enough. Today, however, the term 'supplement' tends to mean anything over-the-counter.

Many supplements are recommended for those who have AI and are taking doctor-prescribed corticosteroids.

Corticosteroids include:

• *Beclomethasome* (Beconase, Beclovent, Vancenase, Vanceril)
• *Budesonide* (Pulmicort, Rhinocort)
• *Dexamethasone* (Decadron, Decadron Phosphate, Turbinaire, and others)
• *Dexamethasone/Tobramycon* (Tobradex)
• *Flunisolide* (AeroBid, Nasaslide)
• *Fluticasone* (Cutivate, Flonase)
• *Hydrocortisone* (Cortef, Hytone, and others)
• *Methylprednisolone* (Medrol and others)
• *Mometasone* (Elocon)
• *Prednisone* (Deltasone, Orasone, and others)
• *Prednisolone* (Delta-cortef, Pediapred, and others)
• *Triamcinolone* (Aristocort, Azmacort, Nasacort, and others)

Depending on your level of AI, various supplements can be recommended in various dosages and frequency. Some persons with CAH produce limited amounts or cortisol, and some produce no or limited aldosterone while others have normal aldosterone levels. Persons with Addison's usually produce no cortisol, and some produce limited aldosterone while others have normal aldosterone levels.

Evaluate the supplements below, and should any of them seem to be what you need, discuss with your practitioner before adding to your daily routine. There may be contraindications with other supplements or medications you are taking, or there may be other factors involved.

Bee Venom

If you are not allergic to bee stings, you may decide to take advantage of bee venom as a supplement.

Used for centuries, bee venom has proven to be an effective and safe treatment for numerous common ailments. Extensive research and clinical work at university centers in Russia, Austria, Germany, France, England, Switzerland, and Czechoslovakia suggests that this therapy may be useful for a number of ailments. However, with AI, the ideal component is the peptide compound it contains called 'melittin.' Melittin stimulates the pituitary-adrenal axis to release both adrenaline and cortisol. (Melittin is also gangliotytic, having the ability to block transmissions of nerve impulses from one cell to another in nerve ganglions, interrupting pain cycles and other central and autonomic nervous system transmissions.)

The components of the bee venom are 11 peptides, 5 enzymes, 3 physiologically active amines, carbohydrates, lipids and amino acids.

CAUTION: *People who have allergic reactions to bee stings should consult a physician before ingesting.*

The concentration of honey/bee venom that would equal 6.5 mg of venom is equal to half a bee sting. The first intake of the honey/bee venom should be without food or drink, in the amount of half a teaspoon, or 0.25 sting. If no allergic reaction occurs, increase the dosage gradually up to 3-4 teaspoons per day. Don't take with food or drink, and keep in mouth until it dissolves.

Vitamin B Complex

Look for products with high levels of vitamin B5 and higher numbers of the rest of the B-complex group, including support nutrients and cofactors. (Dove Health Products has a wonderful product called Vitamin B Complex/Multivitamin: Basic Cell Energy). The recommended dose is 2 daily; 1 in the morning and 1 at noon. Taking it later in the day can interfere with sleep, which is particularly important to keep regular, as cortisol is produced in the 3:00 a.m. vicinity *if* you are sleeping. Start slowly, as tolerated, and build the dose up to the full dose at a rate comfortable for you. A small number of people can only tolerate ½ tablets in the morning and slowly need to build up tolerance to full dose. Dosage may need to be adjusted according to client's weight. Not recommended during pregnancy. If adrenal function improves with this and other dietary and nutritional therapies, or pharmaceutical medications, blood sugar and blood pressure can raise. If these occur to levels that are too high, you may need to recommend a lower dose.

Corticosteroids may increase the loss of Vitamin B6. It is suggested that people taking corticosteroids for longer than 2 weeks should supplement with 25 to 50 mg of Vitamin B6 per day. You should also supplement with B-12 if you take the pharmaceutical Metformin.

If you have any MTHFR mutations, you will want to make sure you have proper forms of methylated B's and folic acids.

Hydrolyzed Collagen

Poor adrenal function is often associated with poor ability to digest protein. Amino acids strengthen the adrenals, and hydrolyzed collagen is a complete source of amino acids. Available as a liquid, it can be mixed with water to improve tolerance of taste. Two tablespoons should be administered during the day. It can be taken at any time throughout the day, with or without food.

Vitamin D

Although the majority of people in the Western world are Vitamin D deficient, this deficiency is almost universal in AI (and other illnesses, including Multiple Sclerosis).

John Cannell, MD, from the Vitamin D Council, asserts that calcitrol, made from D3 when blood values are high enough, "is the most potent steroid hormone in the human body." Vitamin D is actually a hormone, not a vitamin, as well, and individuals need at least 2000-4000 IU/day, or parathyroid hormones remain constantly elevated and absorption of important minerals such as calcium, magnesium and zinc is hindered. These minerals are needed to support the nervous system and deficiencies cause poor stress tolerance, which is exacerbated by AI. Vitamin D deficiency is often a key factor behind poor mineral absorption and once Vitamin D levels are restored and maintained, absorption of these crucial nutrients will improve.

Steroidal anti-inflammatory drugs reduce the body's ability to activate Vitamin D, increasing the risk of bone loss.

A weekly 50,000 IU of Vitamin D3 can help restore Vitamin D levels, with a more regular intake of 2000-4000 IU's per day following repair.

Proline

A dosage of approximately 500 mg each day of Proline can be taken to augment free-form aminos if needed. This will help rebuild connective tissues, and deficient adrenals are often associated with poor quality connective tissues. Any supplement or nutrient that helps connective tissues helps adrenals, as well.

Cordyceps

Cordyceps is a Chinese mushroom that is traditionally used for supporting the adrenals. The *usual dosage is one to two tables, three times a day.*

Pregnenolone

Pregnenolone is a precursor to many adrenal hormones. It is a raw material that supports basic adrenal gland hormone production. It is best taken towards the evening, but if sleep interruption is an issue, the pregnenolone may be taken earlier. The usual dose is 25 mg. It is advisable to have pregnenolone blood levels checked before beginning this supplement. If your levels warrant supplementing, then blood levels should be rechecked and tested at regular intervals.

Digestive Enzymes

Most often, poor adrenal function is also associated with poor digestion and low gastric activity. It is best to use digestive enzymes that contain hydrochloric acid (normally found as Betaine Hydrochloride). 1-2 tablets should be taken during each meal (1, or 2, depending on size of the meal. A normal sized meal would require 1). If you develop acid reflux, it is often because not enough acid is present and the reason for the burning is insufficient protection of the stomach lining. Antacids are the last things you want to take! The persistent heartburn while taking Digestive Enzymes can be relieved by adequate amounts of water, sucking or chewing on deglycyrrhzenized licorice (which will also help what aldosterone levels you have work better, and also contains a glucocorticoid property). Chewing or sucking on the DGL stimulates the production of protective gastric mucus secretions. Slippery Elm, taken 5-30 minutes before a meal, also helps produce protective gastric secretions. Rarely, burning can be assessed by taking digestive acid after several days of building up the mucus lining of the stomach. If there is a burning sensation with the added acid, then there is a good chance that extra acid is not needed, and any burning is not from too much (therefore antacids would be detrimental), but from insufficient stomach lining. To relieve the burning from the assessment, a half-teaspoon of bicarbonate in half a glass of water should relieve the burning. If this is the case, one should not take the additional hydrochloric acid with the digestive enzymes; but instead, only plain digestive enzymes in a minimal dose.

Magnesium

Corticosteroids may increase the loss of magnesium. Some nutritionally oriented doctors recommend that people taking corticosteroids for more than 2 weeks supplement with 300-400 mg of magnesium per day. Magnesium is important for cellular energy (ATP) production. Magnesium Chloride is possibly the most effective form of Magnesium for purposes of cellular detoxification and tissue purification. This form of Magnesium has a strong excretory effect on toxins and stagnant materials stuck in the tissues of the body, drawing them out through the pores of the skin due to the both positive and negative aspects of the electrolytes magnesium and chloride. Chloride is also required to produce a large quantity of gastric acid each day, and is also needed to stimulate starch-digesting enzymes. In addition to functioning as an electrolyte, chloride combines with hydrogen in the stomach to make hydrochloric acid, a powerful digestive enzyme that is responsible for the breakdown of proteins, absorption of other metallic minerals, and activation of intrinsic factors, which in turn, absorbs Vitamin B-12.

Chloride is a highly important and vital mineral required for both human and other animal life, and without chloride, the human body would be unable to maintain fluid in blood vessels (maintains blood volume), conduct nerve transmissions, move muscles, or maintain proper kidney function. Chloride is a major electrolyte mineral of the body, and performs many, many life sustaining roles.

N-Acetyl Cysteine (NAC)

One preliminary study found that adding 600 mg N-acetyl cysteine, or NAC, 3 times per day to treatment with prednisone led to further improvement than with prednisone alone in people with fibrosing alveolitis.

Vitamin A

In some individuals, treatment with corticosteroids can result in impaired wound healing. In one study, topical or internal administration of Vitamin A improved wound healing in eight of ten people on corticosteroid therapy.

GABA

If you suffer from severe panic, anxiety and similar disorders from hormone imbalance, Gamma-aminobutyric acid stimulates GABA receptors, which is what Valium does. The typical effect is decreased anxiety. The usual dose is 500 mg 2 to 3 times per day; start low, increase as needed after assessing after being on the minimum dose for at least 4 weeks.

DHEA

DHEA is a basic adrenal hormone that the adrenal glands will convert into other hormones, including sex hormones. Before starting this supplement (which is actually a prescription in some countries, but not the US) please have DHEA levels checked. If someone is very deficient in this hormone, they may only be able to tolerate a small amount, such as 5 mg. The average adult dose ranges between 10 and 25 mg. The average adult dose ranges between 10 and 25 mg. Start with the minimal dose and have DHEA and cortisol levels checked before raising, to ensure it is working and to assess whether raising is needed, at all. DHEA also goes on the convert to the sex hormones testosterone and estrogen; it is best to avoid it if there is a history of sex organ cancers, such as prostate, uterine or even breast, cervical, testicular, and ovarian.

7-keto DHEA

This form does not convert to sex hormones such as testosterone, but still gives significant support to adrenal functions. The typical dose is 25 mg. each morning, if shown to be warranted through testing.

MSM

MSM is a nutritional form of sulfur and supports connective tissue such as hair, skin, nails, tendons, ligament, bones, etc. Some people do not metabolize sulfur well and cannot take this supplement. The usual dose is 2 to 3 grams daily.

Essential Fatty Acids

These fatty acids are termed 'essential' because our body needs them for good health, but cannot manufacture them. They support the healing process. It may be taken in capsule form or as a liquid; some people use the liquid in cooking. As the vitamins and minerals contained in this are oil soluble, they do not require daily consumption.

Ashwaganda

Ashwaganda is a member of the Solanaceae family and has been used for over 4,000 years in India, Pakistan and Sri Lanka, and as part of Ayurvedic medicine. It is both a tonic and an adaptogen, helping regulate cortisol levels. It is used in the Middle East to help promote normal sleep patterns and encourage a healthy inflammatory response.

Ginseng

There is American Ginseng and Chinese Ginseng; for the adrenal program, Red Panax (Asian) Ginseng is recommended. For background purposes it is worthy to note that Ginseng has been used since time immemorial by Native Americans for debilitating illness, old age, sexual drive, and regulating sleep and body patterns. Today, there is research being done on the effects of American Ginseng and normalizing blood sugar. Ginseng helps the body adapt to stress and normalizes cortisol levels.

Licorice Root

Licorice Root (Clycyrrhiza Glabra and G. Uralensis) offers multiple benefits, along with adrenal support. It has anti-inflammatory and antiviral properties, and can help with digestive, respiratory and urinary infections and irritations. It assists in the healing of ulcers, and may correct many hormonal imbalances but mostly it contains triterpenoid saponins which affect the cortisol balance in the body. Glycyrrhiza Glabra can increase intravascular volume, similar to the medication Fludrocortisone (Florinef) and its action for aldosterone deficiency in salt wasting patients. The normal physiology for sodium-water retention is largely influenced by the expression of mineralocorticoids. While aldosterone is regarded as the main hormone binding to mineralocorticoid receptors involved in the regulation of sodium reabsorption and potassium excretion in the distal renal tubules of the kidney, cortisol also binds to this receptor with the same binding affinity as aldosterone. Interestingly, even though cortisol blood concentrations tend to be greater than aldosterone concentrations, the effect of aldosterone dominates in terms of regulating sodium and water reabsorption and blood volume.

The increased cortisol resulting from licorice use increases gene expression and availability of several enzymes. The first of these is the Na ion permease enzyme which allows for a greater increase in citrate synthase activity within the mitochondria for the purpose of increasing the number of ATP available to fuel the increase in Na/K ATPease activity on the basal-lateral side of the renal tubular cell.

Dosage should not be above 100 mg of supplement, and use of tea should be limited to one cup per day. Nibs, in emergency use, can only be assessed by your noticing any benefits.

In addition to supplements, it is also available in the form of Licorice powder, Licorice tea, or pure Licorice nibs/candy. Please note: American Licorice candy does NOT contain any, or near enough if any at all, amounts of real Licorice. Italian nibs in a tin are excellent to carry for an 'as needed' basis.

Tulsi (Holy Basil)

Tulsi, or Holy Basil, is consumed mostly in supplement form or as Tulsi Tea and is used to treat anxiety, adrenal disorders, hypothyroidism, acne and blood sugar issues.

As far as adrenal issues, it is considered a 'super androgen,' which doesn't affect an individual's mood but helps the body function at its optimal level by modulating the production of cortisol.

Zinc

Zinc deficiency is common in AI. Zinc is an aggressive aromatase inhibitor that will reduce the conversion of testosterone to estrogen in the body. When we don't have enough zinc, levels of the aromatase enzyme rise and the individual will experience a weakened sex drive, reduce muscle mass and increase body fat, among other problems. Zinc is needed for the production of DHEA.

A diet adequate in red meat will provide good quantities of zinc, but with AI, it may be necessary to supplement, and many find that working up slowly reduces the chances of minor side effects. For those individuals who are taking folic acid, folate and iron, it is best to take zinc supplements, or even homeopathic medications like Zicam, approximately an hour separate from the iron related supplements. Have your Zinc levels checked periodically, however, as an overabundance of zinc can lower cortisol.

Marine Plasma

Hypertonic marine plasma can be particularly beneficial to those with low aldosterone/salt wasters. It can restore the electrolyte balance of the body, revitalize body cells, and re-establish biological equilibrium of your body's organisms. It is totally compatible with pharmaceutical prescriptions and over-the-counter drugs. It should be noted that hypertonic marine plasma is not recommended in cases of high blood pressure, or cardiac or kidney problems, where Isotonic Marine Plasma is the best choice.

A total of 83 bioavailable elements in natural seawater at biological temperature, each liter of seawater corresponds on average to 300 milligrams of prebiotic carbon derivatives, such as amino acids, sugars, vitamins, etc. The ions, which are present in liquid form but missing in solid form, are natural chemical and electronic elements that are transformed by the phyto-plankton and zoo-plankton in natural chains. It can be taken per protocols established by the manufacturer of the particular brand you are taking, or in conjunction with a naturopathic practitioner or other practitioner.

Salt Tablets

Salt tablets were the main treatment for low aldosterone/salt wasters for many, many years until Fludrocortisone was approved in the mid 20th century. It is still used today, recommended by both holistic practitioners as a supplement, and by orthodox allopathic physicians (MDs). Salt tablets can be purchased at commercial drug stores, and are often used by athletes, construction workers, truck drivers, etc. They are a good staple item for situations where normal salt intake (normal, meaning additional salt in the salt waster's diet) is depleted due to environment. The recommended dosage is on the packaging, and having established your patterns from your monitoring, you will be able to know when more salt is needed, and when enough supplementation with tablets is enough.

Sole

Sole is an excellent supplement for salt wasters, and can be made at home. More information and a recipe are in Chapter 10 – Hydration.

Things to Beware Of

Beware of any supplements that say they relieve stress! No supplement, oil, music, exercise or anything else can reduce stress, only reduce the *effects* of stress – the stress hormone cortisol! When you are using a product that says it reduces stress, you are actually using something that reduces what little cortisol you may have, or will fight your medication such as hydrocortisone, etc.

There are even weight loss products that are culprits. For example, Corti-Trim purports to reduce stress and bellyfat (targeted bellyfat is a symptom of too much cortisol). As you can tell by the name, it involves cortisol, and in this case, reducing cortisol.

Many stress relieving products contain Lavender, which is also a cortisol reducing compound.

The only way you can relieve stress is to get activities and problems off your plate, or off your radar and eliminate the stressor from your life. This includes physiological stress from your body. When your body is fighting hard and always combatting infections, inflammation, viruses, or the damage of eating hard to digest foods, oils, etc., it also is stress. You have control over what you eat, and how you treat your body. Don't use products that you ingest, inhale, or otherwise get into your system that claim to reduce stress levels!

Chapter Twelve

Daily Care
Treatments

Many people think that alternative medicine is just 'herbs.' Or just 'Homeopathic' medicine, Or just 'Ayurvedic'. You get the drift.

This chapter explains the differences between the more common modalities in alternative medicine. The list below explains the focus of each; it's sort of like in the allopathic (MD, or 'regular' doctors of these days) modality, there are many different types. There are many different types of alternative doctors, too, and in addition to these listed below there are scores more. And each uses hundreds of different specialties within their scope, such as iridology, cupping, sound therapy, body work, reflexology, working in conjunction with regular allopathic medicine, etc.

Here we go:

Complementary And Alternative Medicine (CAM)

It is important to understand the difference between complementary medicine and alternative medicine — the two approaches are often lumped together but are, in fact, distinct.

Complementary medicine refers to healing practices and products that work in conjunction with traditional medicine. For example, a cancer patient receiving chemotherapy may also undergo acupuncture to help manage chemo side effects like nausea and vomiting. Alternative medicine differs in that it is not used as a complement to, but rather as a substitute for traditional therapy. An example would be a cancer patient who forgoes recommended chemotherapy and instead chooses to treat the disease with specific dietary changes.

There is a third category that also often gets lumped in with conventional and alternative medicine — integrative medicine. Integrative medicine draws from both complementary medicine and alternative medicine and combines these with traditional Western therapies, says Donald Abrams, MD, director of clinical programs for the Osher Center for Integrative Medicine at the University of California, San Francisco.

The National Center for Complementary and Alternative Medicine (NCCAM) recently surveyed Americans on their use of complementary and alternative medicine. The survey, which gathered information from more than 20,000 adults and nearly 10,000 children, found that about 40 percent of adults and 12 percent of children use some form of complementary and alternative medicine.
Women, people ages 40 to 60, and adults with higher levels of education and income tended to use complementary and alternative therapies more frequently. There have been considerable increases in the number of people using common forms of complementary and alternative medicine, such as yoga, meditation, acupuncture, and massage therapy.

Many universities, including Georgetown, Rutgers, Duke, and many others have CAM programs. NIH and the Mayo Clinic also have CAM divisions. CAM integrates the forms of alternative medicine shown below, among others.

Ayurveda

Ayurvedic medicine -- also known as Ayurveda -- is one of the world's oldest holistic (whole-body) healing systems. It was developed thousands of years ago in India.

It is based on the belief that health and wellness depend on a delicate balance between the mind, body, and spirit. The primary focus of Ayurvedic medicine is to promote good health, rather than fight disease. But treatments may be recommended for specific health problems. Herbs and nutrition/diet are a large part of the non-spiritual side of Ayurvedic medicine, and numerous commercial products are available that are 'ayurvedic,' particularly from India.

Traditional Chinese Medicine (TCM)

The current name for an ancient system of health care from China. Traditional Chinese medicine (TCM) is based on a concept of balanced qi (pronounced "chee"), or vital energy, that is believed to flow throughout the body. Qi is proposed to regulate a person's spiritual, emotional, mental, and physical balance and to be influenced by the opposing forces of yin (negative energy) and yang (positive energy). Disease is proposed to result from the flow of qi being disrupted and yin and yang becoming imbalanced. Among the components of TCM are herbal and nutritional therapy, restorative physical exercises, meditation, acupuncture, and remedial massage.

Chiropractic
Chiropractic is a health care profession that focuses on disorders of the musculoskeletal system and the nervous system, and the effects of these disorders on general health. Chiropractic care is used most often to treat neuromusculoskeletal complaints, including but not limited to back pain, neck pain, pain in the joints of the arms or legs, and headaches, but the nerves connected to the spinal system affect many bodily functions.

Doctors of Chiropractic – often referred to as chiropractors or chiropractic physicians – practice a drug-free, hands-on approach to health care that includes patient examination, diagnosis and treatment. Chiropractors have broad diagnostic skills and are also trained to recommend therapeutic and rehabilitative exercises, as well as to provide nutritional, dietary and lifestyle counseling.

The most common therapeutic procedure performed by doctors of chiropractic is known as "spinal manipulation," also called "chiropractic adjustment." The purpose of manipulation is to restore joint mobility by manually applying a controlled force into joints that have become hypomobile – or restricted in their movement – as a result of a tissue injury. Tissue injury can be caused by a single traumatic event, such as improper lifting of a heavy object, or through repetitive stresses, such as sitting in an awkward position with poor spinal posture for an extended period of time. In either case, injured tissues undergo physical and chemical changes that can cause inflammation, pain, and diminished function for the sufferer. Manipulation, or adjustment of the affected joint and tissues, restores mobility, thereby alleviating pain and muscle tightness, and allowing tissues to heal.

Doctors of chiropractic may assess patients through clinical examination, laboratory testing, diagnostic imaging and other diagnostic interventions to determine when chiropractic treatment is appropriate or when it is not appropriate. Many Chiropractors are also certified, licensed and practice other alternative modalities, such as Naturopathy, Homeopathy, Nutrition, etc., and Chiropractors will readily refer patients to the appropriate health care provider when chiropractic care is not suitable for the patient's condition, or the condition warrants co-management in conjunction with other members of the health care team, as do most practitioners involved in Complementary and Alternative Medicine (CAM).

Herbalism/Herbology

Herbal medicine -- also called botanical medicine or phytomedicine -- refers to using a plant's seeds, berries, roots, leaves, bark, or flowers for medicinal purposes. Herbalism has a long tradition of use outside of conventional medicine. It is becoming more mainstream as improvements in analysis and quality control along with advances in clinical research show the value of herbal medicine in the treating and preventing disease. Herbalism is the common terminology for this practice, and Herbology is the common phrase for those who share their knowledge of herbs from either cultural, folklore, or familial sources or self learning.

Holistic Medicine

Holistic Medicine is a form of healing that considers the whole person -- body, mind, spirit, and emotions -- in the quest for optimal health and wellness. According to the holistic medicine philosophy, one can achieve optimal health -- the primary goal of holistic medicine practice -- by gaining proper balance in life.

Holistic medicine practitioners believe that the whole person is made up of interdependent parts and if one part is not working properly, all the other parts will be affected. In this way, if people have imbalances (physical, emotional, or spiritual) in their lives, it can negatively affect their overall health.

A holistic doctor may use all forms of health care, from conventional medication to alternative therapies, to treat a patient. For example, when a person suffering from migraine headaches pays a visit to a holistic doctor, instead of walking out solely with medication, the doctor will likely take a look at all the potential factors that may be causing the person's headaches, such as other health problems, diet and sleep habits, stress and personal problems, and preferred spiritual practices. The treatment plan may involve drugs to relieve symptoms, but also lifestyle modifications to help prevent the headaches from recurring.

Holistic Nutrition

Holistic Nutrition is a professional trained in Natural Nutrition and complementary therapies, whose principal function is to educate individuals and groups about the benefits and health impact of optimal nutrition.

Mainstream medicine does not emphasize the significance of improper nutrition as a major cause of a wide range of health disorders. Although most people are aware of the benefits of sound nutrition, the range of conflicting information available to the consumer is often confusing. Holistic nutritionists guide their clients through the maze of information. They work with clients to identify and help correct the nutritional causes of diseases, illnesses and injuries, and they are qualified to design personalized diet and lifestyle programs that optimize the clients' concerns and health.

Homeopathy

Homeopathy, or homeopathic medicine, is a medical philosophy and practice based on the idea that the body has the ability to heal itself. Homeopathy was founded in the late 1700s in Germany and has been widely practiced throughout Europe. Homeopathic medicine views symptoms of illness as normal responses of the body as it attempts to regain health.

Homeopathy is based on the idea that "like cures like." That is, if a substance causes a symptom in a healthy person, giving the person a very small amount of the same substance may cure the illness. In theory, a homeopathic dose of chemically compounded homeopathic medicines, enhances the body's normal healing and self-regulatory processes.

A homeopathic health practitioner (homeopath) uses these pills or liquid mixtures (solutions) containing only a little of an active ingredient (usually a plant or mineral) for treatment of disease. These are known as highly diluted or "potentiated" substances.

Indigenous Medicine

Indigenous Medicine encompasses the traditional healing practices of any culture. Native American, Aborigine, etc. Each culture has different treatments and philosophies, and are commonly used by these indigenous communities. In the case of Native Americans, laws allow traditional healers to work with allopathic physicians and hospitals to treat federally recognized tribal citizens.

Naturopathic

Naturopathic medicine is a distinct primary health care profession, emphasizing prevention, treatment, and optimal health through the use of therapeutic methods and substances that encourage individuals' inherent self-healing process. The practice of naturopathic medicine includes modern and traditional, scientific, and empirical methods. The following principles are the foundation of naturopathic medical practice:

• <u>The Healing Power of Nature</u> (Vis Medicatrix Naturae): Naturopathic medicine recognizes an inherent self-healing process in people that is ordered and intelligent. Naturopathic physicians act to identify and remove obstacles to healing and recovery, and to facilitate and augment this inherent self-healing process.
• <u>Identify and Treat the Causes</u> (Tolle Causam): The naturopathic physician seeks to identify and remove the underlying causes of illness rather than to merely eliminate or suppress symptoms.
• <u>First Do No Harm</u> (Primum Non Nocere): Naturopathic physicians follow three guidelines to avoid harming the patient:
◦ Utilize methods and medicinal substances which minimize the risk of harmful side effects, using the least force necessary to diagnose and treat;
◦ Avoid when possible the harmful suppression of symptoms; and
◦ Acknowledge, respect, and work with individuals' self-healing process.
• <u>Doctor as Teacher</u> (Docere): Naturopathic physicians educate their patients and encourage self-responsibility for health. They also recognize and employ the therapeutic potential of the doctor-patient relationship.
• <u>Treat the Whole Person</u>: Naturopathic physicians treat each patient by taking into account individual physical, mental, emotional, genetic, environmental, social, and other factors. Since total health also includes spiritual health, naturopathic physicians encourage individuals to pursue their personal spiritual development.
• <u>Prevention</u>: Naturopathic physicians emphasize the prevention of disease by assessing risk factors, heredity and susceptibility to

disease, and by making appropriate interventions in partnership with their patients to prevent illness.

Naturopathic practice includes the following diagnostic and therapeutic modalities: clinical and laboratory diagnostic testing, nutritional medicine, botanical medicine, naturopathic physical medicine (including naturopathic manipulative therapy), public health measures, hygiene, counseling, minor surgery, homeopathy, acupuncture, prescription medication, intravenous and injection therapy, and naturopathic obstetrics (natural childbirth).

Osteopathy

DOs and MDs are Alike in Many Ways.
• Students entering both DO and MD medical colleges typically have already completed four-year bachelor's degrees with an emphasis on scientific courses.
• Both DOs and MDs complete four years of medical school.
• After medical school, both DOs and MDs obtain graduate medical education through internships, residencies and fellowships. This training lasts three to eight years and prepares DOs and MDs to practice a specialty.
• Both DOs and MDs can choose to practice in any specialty of medicine—such as pediatrics, family medicine, psychiatry, surgery or ophthalmology.
• DOs and MDs must pass comparable examinations to obtain state licenses.
• DOs and MDs both practice in accredited and licensed health care facilities.
• Together, DOs and MDs enhance the state of health care available in the U.S.

While DOs and MDs have many things in common, osteopathic medicine is a parallel branch of American medicine with a distinct philosophy and approach to patient care. DOs can bring an extra dimension to your health care through their unique skills. For more than a century, osteopathic physicians have built a tradition of bringing health care to where it is needed most:

• Approximately 60% of practicing osteopathic physicians practice in the primary care specialties of family medicine, general internal medicine, pediatrics, and obstetrics and gynecology.

• Many DOs fill a critical need for physicians by practicing in rural and other medically underserved communities.

In addition, these modern-day pioneers practice on the cutting edge of medicine. DOs combine today's medical technology with their ears to listen caringly to their patients, with their eyes to see each patient as a whole person, and with their hands to diagnose and treat patients for injury and illness.

As stated, there are many sub-types and specialties within these modalities, but they all are what is considered 'alternative.' Alternative to what? Alternative to Western (allopathic, or MD's) which have only been around for about 100 years? Indeed, Allopathic, when compared with treatments and philosophies over the years, and compared to treatments and philosophies around the world, is truly the 'alternative,' but alas, ancient and still widely used methods are considered 'alternative' just because they are not the norm in the mid to late 20th century, but that is changing in the early 21st century.

Following are a few alternative treatments that may be useful to the AI patient. There are many treatments available to help you specific to each above modality, but these are a few good treatments you should be able to locate a practitioner for, or provide the treatment yourself.

Ultrasound Therapy

Ultrasound therapy is a method of stimulating cells that are beneath the skin's surface. Cells, as you know, are the very building blocks of life. Ultrasound uses extremely high frequencies that cannot by heard by humans, between 800,000 Hz and 2,000,000 Hz.

While this therapy is often used to break up stony deposits or accelerate the effect of drugs in certain areas, it can be particularly helpful in the AI patient who is experiencing Third Spacing. This is when the patient has enough fluids, but electrolytes are not moving them through the cells and they are just 'sitting' in interstitial places. Then you become dehydrated as the fluids are not being used. If you are dehydrated, your blood pressure is dropping, and you feel like trouble may be coming, in addition to updosing, often taking marine plasma, electrolytes or salt (tablets or table) and using ultrasound on your abdomen, the sides of your face in front of your ear (near the parotid gland), can help get fluids moving again. Home ultrasound units are available which are not strong enough for major procedures, but are certainly enough for this procedure. Use the wand for 3 minutes on each area.

Acupuncture

Acupuncture can be an extremely effective modality to treat many symptoms. One thing to remember is that while there is no specific point for AI, there are points that address the myriad of symptoms. However, *any* acupuncture point and procedure stimulates the adrenals.

Acupuncture has been around for thousands of years, and is a common practice in Eastern countries, while large corporation even have acupuncturists on staff to treat employees.

Acupuncture focuses on the flow of energy, or *chi* in the body, and influences the activity of adenosine which is an amino acid which becomes active in the skin after injury to ease pain. This reaches all areas of your body, not just the point where the painless needle is inserted. There are many subtle actions that take place depending on where the needle is placed, but most important is the flow of energy, almost like a system of invisible nerves, that takes place. It is a way to treat many symptoms of AI or other symptoms that could be stressing your body, without the use of harmful pharmaceuticals which could produce other side effects and stresses on the body.

A good practitioner, or even a Chinese doctor should you be so lucky to live in an area where there are Chinese doctors in practice, can be an important member of your team when you have pain, healing from an injury, or even want to treat chronic maladies or even stop smoking or put hot flashes at bay!

It is harmless and there are no known side effects from acupuncture; however, if you experience anything unusual, please contact your physician or primary practitioner.

Mineral Baths

Not all salts are 'salt' as we commonly think of it. "Salt," as we know it, which is technically Sodium Chloride. There are many 'salts' other than sodium chloride, however.

Mineral baths are used for a variety of reasons, most commonly Epsom Salt baths. Epsom Salt is actually Magnesium Sulfate, not Sodium Chloride. Epsom Salt, named for a bitter saline spring at Epsom in Surrey, England, is a naturally occurring pure mineral compound of magnesium and sulfate. Long known as a natural remedy for a number of ailments, Epsom salt has numerous health benefits as well as many beauty, household and gardening-related uses.

If your memory of high school chemistry is lacking or faded, here is a run-down of Mineral Salts and their uses as therapeutic baths.

Epsom Salt (Magnesium Sulfate). Magnesium sulfate (or magnesium sulphate) is an inorganic salt (chemical compound) containing magnesium, sulfur and oxygen, with the formula $MgSO_4$. It is often encountered as the heptahydrate sulfate mineral epsomite ($MgSO_4 \cdot 7H_2O$), commonly called Epsom Salt. Studies have shown that magnesium and sulfate are both readily absorbed through the skin, making Epsom salt baths an easy and ideal way to enjoy the amazing health benefits . Magnesium plays a number of roles in the body including regulating the activity of over 325 enzymes, makes insulin more effective, reducing inflammation, helping muscle and nerve function and helping to prevent artery hardening. Sulfates help improve the absorption of nutrients, flush toxins and help ease migraine headaches. The importance of Magnesium as an electrolyte and as needing supplementation to those on supplemental cortisol has been covered throughout this book.

Dead Sea Salts. Dead Sea salts have only a fraction of the sodium that table salt has – 12-18% compared to 97%. Dead Sea Salt also contains Chloride and Bromide, Magnesium, Calcium and Potassium, in addition to Sodium. These minerals occur naturally in our bodies and are vital to our overall health. Dead Sea salts are harvested from the Dead Sea, a mineral-rich body of water located between Jordan and Israel. Dead Sea salts carry many benefits, particularly when used as bath salts. Dead Sea salts effectively treat many skin conditions, including from rashes and psoriasis to more everyday conditions such as oily or dry skin. Dead Sea salts are also known to soothe rashes, calm allergic reactions, minimize dandruff and treat acne. Dead Sea salts have been known to improve the appearance of cellulite, manage the appearance of swelling due to water retention, and even treat hair loss. In addition, Dead Sea salts detoxify your skin, drawing out dirt, pollutants and impurities from each pore.

There is nothing more calming than a bath with Dead Sea salts; the minerals in Dead Sea salts, when combined with warm water, work to increase your circulation while decreasing your heart rate, reducing anxiety and stress. Many swear by Dead Sea salts as an effective treatment for insomnia and other sleep disorders.

Himalayan Salt. Himalayan salts are considered the most pure salts in the world, and contain upwards of 84 minerals. Himalayan salt contains the minerals that are necessary for your health, including macrominerals and trace minerals. The macrominerals are needed in relative abundance and include calcium, chloride, iron, magnesium, phosphorus, potassium and sodium. The recommended daily amount of these macrominerals depends of your age, activity level and general health. Calcium is the most common mineral in your body and is found in your bones and teeth, as well as playing a vital role in nerve and muscle health. Trace minerals are needed in small amounts for health, and those found in Himalayan salt include boron, chromium, copper, fluoride, iodine, manganese, molybdenum, selenium and zinc. Other minerals in Himalayan salt include aluminum, carbon, platinum, selenium, sulfur and titanium. In addition to being used as a bath salt, Himalayan salts are quite healthy and used in place of ordinary table salt due to their rich nutrient and mineral content.

Himalayan salts are known to cleanse and detoxify the skin, leaving it smoother, softer, and cleaner than ever before. The numerous minerals and nutrients found in Himalayan salts are released as they are mixed with warm water, and this solution is often referred to as "sole" or "brine water".

Himalayan Salts are an effective treatment for common skin conditions such as dry skin, psoriasis, and acne. They can also be used to soothe insect bites, heal blisters, and even treat ailments that affect our joints, such as arthritis. If you suffer from premenstrual symptoms, a nice warm bath with Himalayan salts can calm your cramps and relieve the pressure and bloating associated with excess water retention. And if you have a difficult time getting to sleep, bathing with Himalayan salts can reduce stress and promote a better night's sleep. When bathing with Himalayan salt, don't be shy about how much you use – the higher the concentration of Himalayan salt in the water, the more beneficial your bath will be.

For those choosing to bathe with healing salts, remember to take your condition and your plan into consideration. For example, if you have a low heart rate, you wouldn't want to use Dead Sea Salts at that particular time, as it is known to lower heart rate.

A Tried and True Detox Bath

1 cup Epsom Salts
1 regular/small box Baking Soda
1 Tablespoon Ground Ginger

Diluted in warm bath.

Bathe for less than 30 minutes to detox, and over 45 minutes if you wish to absorb the nutrients.

Chapter Thirteen

Daily Care
In Case of Emergency

As much as we all hate the thought of an emergency, more than likely we will all experience one or more during our lives. As an AI patient, emergencies for others can quickly become an emergency for you, too, as the sudden stress can use up all of your cortisol at an unexpected time when you have not had the opportunity to updose in advance. Sometimes, you may encounter an emergency situation where you are not able to interact with emergency personnel, due to being unconscious or in an adrenal crisis. Or, you may be sent to emergency treatment in an area or facility unfamiliar with you, and with AI.

First and foremost, you should always wear a medical alert bracelet or necklace. Simple bracelets that state your condition only are better than nothing, but since so many EMS services and Emergency Rooms do not have protocols for AI, you should attempt to use a product which is more informative and helpful.

Emergency personnel I have interviewed state that they prefer bracelets over necklaces or even tattoos, because they are much easier to identify as a 'medical alert.' Some people have numerous tattoos and it is difficult to locate a medical tattoo amongst them. There are bracelets available that have a compartment that opens where you can place folded paperwork such as instructions for treatment, emergency contacts, and your physicians contact details. These are the most helpful. There are also high-tech ones available that carry an ID number, for example, where the emergency personnel can log into the service and find all of your information, records, and more (whatever you have uploaded). However, personnel state that it is not feasible many times for them to log in and search for such info.

As stated earlier in this book, personnel are trained on how to react if the ID says "Adrenal Insufficiency" or "Steroid Dependent." "Addison's Disease" is not always recognizable, and if the responder is looking up protocols in a database, it is usually listed as "Adrenal Insufficiency." In any event, 'steroid dependent' is understood by most. They know you can't stop cold turkey and it is important to make sure you have your steroids, particularly when in a trauma situation. They can find out the exact details of your condition later.

You should always carry an emergency injection, marked with your name and instructions. If you are unconscious, it is helpful for responders to know that this is, indeed, *your* injection and when it should be administered. If you should need the injection while away from home , it is easily available by yourself, or whomever is with you. Try to always carry it in the same location so people can find it, or you can remember where it is when you are having cognitive dysfunction. Like 'in the side pocket of my purse,' or something similar.

There are a multitude of other identifiers available you may wish to consider based on your circumstances. There are wraps for seat belts in the event you are in an accident. These usually state "Adrenal Insufficiency – steroid dependent," etc. There are special bags for your injection and meds, magnets for your car door, bumper stickers, etc. All of them have been blessings for people out there who were saved through quick intervention due to these items.

An ICE, or "In Case of Emergency" app or wallpaper on your phone is an excellent idea. Personnel I interviewed stated that they look for these much more often than emergency contact cards in wallets today. Make sure that the one you use is accessible without cell service or internet so it can be accessed anywhere, anytime, and make sure it can be accessed without putting a PIN in your phone. If your phone unlocks with your fingerprint, emergency personnel aren't always authorized to use an unconscious person's fingerprint without their knowledge, so another reason to make sure it's accessible. A screen shot as wallpaper is a good alternative to make sure it is seen.

Emergency Letters are becoming more and more popular. There are horror stories each and every day of AI patients having a crisis who are denied intervention by either uninformed and untrained personnel, or staff at Emergency Rooms who think it is 'ok' to wait until your GP or endocrinologist make an appearance at the hospital. This has led to organ failure and damage, disabilities, hospitals and staff being sued, and even death.

On the next page is verbiage that can be used to create your own letter for your endocrinologist to sign. Have one on file at your local hospital, with your GP, and carry copies with you and even one in your glovebox, and a photo of one uploaded to your ICE app, if possible. You may also want to fill it out in this book and keep the book with you, so that in an emergency, others will have a well-rounded source of information.

ADRENAL INSUFFICIENCY • URGENT

Name:

Address:

Date of Birth:

Endocrinologist:

Primary Care Physician:

Medical Condition:

To Whom it May Concern:

The person named in this letter has a medical condition which is classified as Adrenal Insufficiency which results in cortisol dependency due to insufficient cortisol. When this person is in an accident or seriously ill, it is imperative that this be treated as a medical emergency, and a life threatening Adrenal Crisis (or Addisonian Crisis) can quickly occur without intervention.

Solu-Cortef, or other glucocorticoid, must be administered through IM injection IMMEDIATELY.

Adrenal crisis occurs when electrolyte imbalances are developed through illness, trauma or accidents, as well. **Please treat with Sodium Chloride IV.**

Signs of an impending Adrenal Crisis can include failure to respond, weakness, dizziness, confusion, nausea, vomiting, hypotension, hypoglycemia, paleness, and cold and clammy to the touch.

100

This patient must be taken to a hospital immediately after receiving such injection.

This patient has an injection on their person to inject. (Do not type this line, or cross out, if not applicable).

This patient must be seen by a physician immediately, and waiting for treatment is inappropriate and life threatening. Contact their Primary Physician or Endocrinologist immediately upon beginning treatment.

Signed:

Printed Name:

Emergency Number:

Chapter Fourteen

Resources

There are many sources for information, but not all of them good, or accurate. Especially in the age of millions of "Google Doctors", forums on social networking, and 'Adrenal Fatigue' blogs. The following are reputable sites to give you more information on· Alternative Health, as well as Adrenal Insufficiency. Remember that each one will have loads of resources and links to other information they feel appropriate.

Alternative Health

National Institute of Health, National Center for Complementary and Integrative Health – www.nccih.nih.gov

Duke University Integrative Medicine – www.dukeintegrativemedicine.org

Adrenal Insufficiency

Adrenal Insufficiency United (Numerous resources and helpful information) – www.aiunited.org

National Adrenal Diseases Foundation (NADF) – www.nadf.us

CAH Is Us (Congenital Adrenal Hyperplasia focused) – www.cahisus.co.uk

CARES Foundation (Congenital Adrenal Hyperplasia focused) – www.caresfoundation.org

National Organization for Rare Diseases (NORD) – www.rarediseases.org

Adrenoleukodystrophy Foundation (ALD) – www.aldfoundation.org

• • • • •

Made in the USA
Middletown, DE
01 September 2023